# THE NON-SURGICAL SKIN REVOLUTION

This book is intended for reference and information only. The advice herein is not intended to replace the services of trained professionals, or to be a substitute for medical advice. You are advised to consult with an accredited professional regarding matters relating to your health, and in particular matters that may require diagnosis or medical attention. The author cannot be held responsible for the outcome of any treatments described in this book or any loss arising from use of this book.

By Sandy Hamber

Copyright © Sandy Hamber 2024
First published December 2024

The right of Sandy Hamber to be identified as the Author of the Work has been asserted by her in accordance with the Copyright, Design and Patents Act 1998.

All rights reserved. This book is copyright material and must not be copied, reproduced, transferred, distributed, leased, licensed or publicly performed or used in any way except as specifically permitted in writing by the author, as allowed under the terms and conditions under which it was purchased or as strictly permitted by applicable copyright law. Any unauthorised distribution or use of this text may be a direct infringement of the author's rights and those responsible may be liable in law accordingly.

Edited by: Ellie Smith
Cover and book design by Nicola Acketts
*foursisters.co.uk*

ISBN: 9798303510883

A Beauty Studio Medi Spa production
bsmedispa.co.uk

# THE NON-SURGICAL SKIN REVOLUTION

**Your ultimate guide to ageing well
– *without* surgery**

By Sandy Hamber

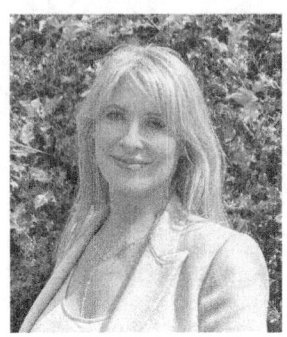

## About the author

I'm Sandy. With over 35 years' experience in the beauty industry, I've witnessed first-hand the evolution of age-defying aesthetic technologies.

Wind back the clock to the 1980s, and beauty treatments were simple. I started my salon aged 21 with nothing but a wax pot, a few tubs of face cream, a second-hand Slendertone machine, a G5 massager, a vacuum suction machine, and a few manicure and pedicure tools. Clients came for waxes, facials, pedicures, and massages, all performed with the straightforward products and tools I had at hand.

Today, my award-winning MediSpa looks very different. I offer the very latest, high-tech, research-supported treatments with the power to transform how we look and feel as we age. I'm thrilled to say that some of my clients have been with me since the very start. One client, Beryl, hasn't missed her monthly manicure, pedicure, and Clarins facial for 35 years. She's just celebrated her 97th birthday and is a testament to the benefits of regular self-care, remaining mentally and physically agile.

We're living in an era of unprecedented access to the best beauty technology. It's never been easier to safely stave off signs of ageing but, for the uninitiated, the sheer number of treatments on offer – each promising to tighten, tone and transform – can be overwhelming. That's why I've written this book. In the following pages, I'll be sharing my experience and expertise to help empower you to make the best decisions for your body, embrace your ageing journey and live life to the fullest.

Enjoy!

Sandy

PS. Connect with me on Instagram *@thebeautystudiomedispa* to see the treatments described in this book in action.

# CONTENTS

11 Introduction: The reason you're holding this book

13 Can I age gracefully without going under the scalpel?

17 What does it mean to age well?

## Part One: *It starts at home*

19 Think yourself younger

24 The science of skin ageing

27 The M word: menopause and your skin

31 The gut-skin connection

35 Am I drinking enough water?

38 Sweet talk: the truth about sugar

40 You booze, you lose

44 Why am I ageing faster than my friends?

46 Smart skincare

54 Beauty sleep

# Part Two: *Find your fix*

| | |
|---|---|
| 58 | Turkey neck |
| 62 | Frown lines |
| 65 | Nose-to-mouth lines |
| 68 | Marionette lines |
| 71 | Double chin |
| 74 | Drooping jowls |
| 78 | Hooded lids |
| 81 | Dark under-eye circles |
| 84 | Under-eye bags |
| 88 | Temporal veins |
| 90 | Lip lines |
| 93 | Crow's feet |
| 96 | Skin tone changes |
| 100 | Age spots and pigmentation |
| 105 | Facial flushing and redness |
| 108 | Common age-related skin blemishes |
| | - Seborrheic keratosis |
| | - Skin tags |
| | - Actinic keratosis |
| | - Lines and wrinkles |
| 111 | Visible pores |
| 114 | Ageing hands |

## Part three: *Your non-surgical journey*

**118**    How to choose a good clinic

**120**    Watch out for perception drift

**123**    Navigating aesthetic treatments after cancer

**125**    Looking ahead to your skincare journey

## Part four: *Treatment index*

**128**    Skin peels

**131**    Radiofrequency

**133**    Fractional radiofrequency

**136**    High-intensity focused ultrasound (HIFU)

         - Micro-focused ultrasound

**139**    Parallel beam ultrasound (Sofwave™)

**141**    High-intensity facial electromagnetic stimulation (HIFES)

**143**    Laser

         - Non-ablative lasers

         - Fractional lasers

         - Ablative lasers

**150**    Intense pulsed light (IPL)

| | |
|---|---|
| **153** | Microneedling |
| | - MesoFacial |
| **156** | Exosomes |
| **158** | Platelet-rich plasma therapy (PRP) |
| **160** | Fat-busting treatments |
| | - Lipolysis injections |
| | - Cryolipolysis ('fat freezing') |
| **164** | Wet microdermabrasion (HydraFacial) |
| **167** | Injectable skin-boosters |
| | - Polynucleotide injections |
| | - Hyaluronic acid injections (injectable moisturisers) |
| **170** | Toxin injections (Botox) |
| **174** | Fillers |
| | - Hyaluronic acid filler |
| | - Calcium hydroxylapatite filler |
| | - Poly-L-lactic acid filler |
| **179** | LED light therapy |
| **182** | Facial thread lifts |
| **190** | Permanent makeup |

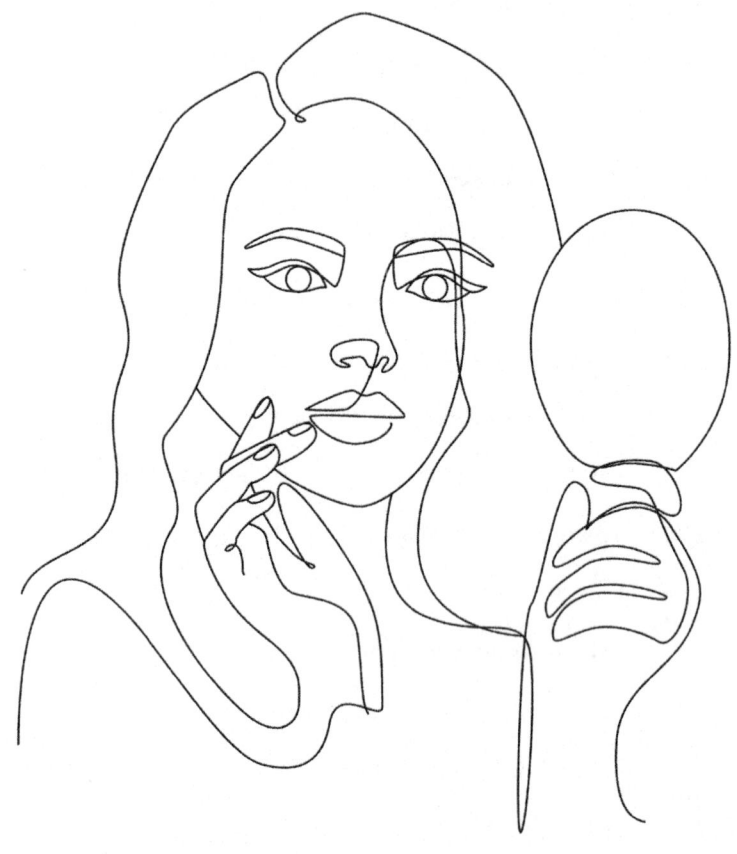

# INTRODUCTION

# The reason you're holding this book

Ageing is a privilege, but it doesn't always feel like one.

In my clinic, I speak to women every day who are struggling with their changing bodies. They tell me they don't recognise the face looking back at them in the mirror and feel far more full of life than their reflection lets on.

Many are repeatedly told they look exhausted, even when they don't feel tired, and tell me that these persistent comments are chipping away at their self-esteem. Others notice a dramatic acceleration of skin ageing during menopause and land in my clinic looking to hit the brakes and maybe even put the ageing process into reverse.

I've helped clients look and feel their best through the very best of times – think anniversaries, weddings and significant birthdays. I've also held their hands through the worst, including the skin and hair changes that come during periods of illness or following cancer treatment.

And let's not forget the curious – the women that find me because they've seen their friend, colleague or family member glowing with confidence and want to know the secret sauce.

So, whatever has led you to pick up this book – whether you're struggling with self-confidence or are simply curious – you're in safe hands. In the following pages, I'll arm you with all the latest evidence-based information you need to safely look and feel your very best for the long haul.

I'll also be encouraging you to embrace ageing as a natural process that should be celebrated. That's why I always use the term 'ageing well' over 'anti-ageing'. We'll look at how you can cultivate better habits that reshape your perception of 'getting on' into something more empowering. There's no reason why the second half of your life can't be the better half. By nourishing our bodies with good food, embracing a fulfilling lifestyle, and dedicating time to personal growth and self-care, we can (and will!) age well.

# Can I age gracefully without going under the scalpel?

Yes, without a doubt. This is what the non-surgical skin revolution is all about!

I've witnessed first-hand how clients – through consistent skincare routines and regular, non-invasive treatments (which I'll detail in upcoming chapters) – have undergone remarkable transformations. In fact, these transformations can be so impressive that clients have a difficult job convincing family and friends that there's been no surgery involved.

But it's important to manage our expectations, too. There's no Benjamin Button-esque magic wand and we can't make time stand still. Results depend on where you are on the ageing spectrum and whether you've had previous interventions.

That said, you don't need to have been a skincare saint since your early twenties to benefit. With advancements in minimally invasive technology and the guidance I'll be sharing in this book, significant improvements are very much within reach.

I'm proof of that. Now aged 56 and, naturally fair-skinned, I've battled the effects of excessive sun exposure – along with horrifying thoughts about the sunbed I used to rent and enjoy in my bedroom. Through diligent care and embracing advancing technologies, I've managed to stave off the signs of ageing to a more reasonable extent than I ever thought possible. As I approach sixty, I feel more confident and comfortable in my own skin than ever before.

## Is surgery ever the answer?

Before continuing, I want to make my stance on cosmetic surgery clear. I'm not against the idea of a facelift. Should there come a time when I'm genuinely discontent with how I'm ageing, and if the array of non-surgical treatments at my disposal cannot meet my expectations, I may entertain the notion of surgery.

But, in my experience, there is rarely an occasion when non-surgical treatments can't help us feel fantastic as we age. This was the case for a client of mine, a vibrant 60-year-old woman, who wanted to reduce the fat below her chin and improve definition along her jawline.

She assumed she'd need a surgical facelift and so consulted a plastic surgeon. Luckily, my client chose a trustworthy surgeon who recommended that she first explore skincare products, as well as safer non-invasive therapies.

Heeding this advice, we embarked on a journey together, with the aim of minimising her 'double chin' and tightening the skin and muscles on her lower face. To achieve this, I used a combination of high-intensity facial electromagnetic stimulation with radio frequency technology. The transformation was considerable, and she was delighted with the outcomes. "I'm so pleased with the result," she said at the time. "It has saved me the expense and the risks associated with surgery." (See the post from July 7th, 2024, on my Instagram page to marvel at the results yourself.)

This story demonstrates the importance of exploring all avenues before settling on surgery. By taking a step back and evaluating all available options, we make the decisions that best align with our wellbeing and aesthetic goals.

## Cosmetic surgery – the risks

Surgery can deliver great results but comes with risks that shouldn't be overlooked. This is why a trustworthy surgeon will always encourage patients to consider less invasive treatment before going under the knife.

Top of the list is the risk of infection. Even with the most stringent sterilisation techniques, the introduction of instruments into the body can lead to infection. If the infection is severe, it can prolong recovery times and, in some cases, lead to more significant health issues.

Then there's anaesthesia to consider. This is required for most surgical procedures and carries its own risks. Complications can range from minor, such as nausea and dizziness, to more severe, including allergic reactions or worse.

Patients can also experience adverse reactions to medications used during or after surgery. Again, these can range from mild allergic reactions to severe side effects that impact recovery and overall health.

Finally, let's not forget the risk of a bad aesthetic outcome. My biggest fear when it comes to surgery is not achieving the look I'd hoped for or, worse, looking in the mirror and not seeing 'me' anymore. While a skilled surgeon can enhance your features, there's always a chance of unexpected results that cannot be reversed. I've seen several clients over the years understandably unhappy with the outcome of their surgery and, even after going back for a second operation, they remain disappointed.

I'm not sharing these risks to scare you. If you do decide that surgery is right for you, it's important to go in with your eyes wide open, weighing up the potential complications and risks with the expected rewards.

## Is surgery right for me?

Risks aside, here are the other factors to consider when deciding whether cosmetic surgery is right for you.

**Time commitment:** Chances are your busy schedule will need adjusting to accommodate time for post-surgical recuperation. The recovery time can vary depending on how invasive the procedure is, as well as your individual capacity for healing. While advancements in surgical techniques have minimised downtime, you should still expect time away from work and other commitments. It's also important to diligently follow post-operative care instructions which can be time-consuming.

**Maintenance:** Surgical procedures can deliver dramatic results, but these results don't necessarily last forever. As the ageing process continues, additional surgeries may be required to sustain the desired outcome. For this reason, it's important to understand the investment of time and money that may be required in the future before undergoing cosmetic surgery. Despite what many believe, surgery is rarely a 'forever' solution.

**Your health:** Not everyone is a suitable candidate for surgery. Certain conditions such as obesity, diabetes, high blood pressure, heart disease, bleeding disorders or poor mental health can increase the likelihood of adverse effects. As can lifestyle factors such as smoking or excessive drinking. A combination of these factors may make surgery a less favourable option for you.

# What does it mean to age well?

I've noticed that women tend to feel the pressure to age gracefully more acutely than men. As writer and midlife champion Eleanor Mills puts it, "we live in a culture which glorifies youth, where men are seen to age like fine wine while women are seen as more like peaches – one wrinkle and we're done."

Yet, when women (especially those in the public eye) take steps to minimise signs of ageing with surgical or non-surgical treatments, they're often accused of vanity and criticised for not taking a more natural approach.

It seems to me that, as women, we're caught between a rock and a hard place when it comes to ageing – we're damned if we do, damned if we don't.

For this reason, I encourage clients to tune out the opinions of others, focusing instead on their own wellbeing and desires. We know that how we look (and crucially, how we *feel* about how we look) has a huge impact on our mood, confidence and how we move through the world.

Research suggests that people who feel good about how they look tend to have more confidence and better self-esteem. They're also generally more comfortable in social situations, leading to enhanced relationships and interactions with others. And, if that wasn't enough, feeling positive about our body has been linked to greater happiness and life satisfaction.

On the other hand, studies suggest that, if we're not confident in our appearance, we're likely to experience higher levels of psychological stress. I've not met one woman who needs more stress in her life.

The beauty industry is waking up to this important connection between how we feel and how we look, with new treatments increasingly embracing a more holistic approach. It's no longer just about looking good but also feeling good. Alongside Botox and filler, you're now likely to find wellness and self-care offerings in your local clinic – from aromatherapy to nutritional advice and mindfulness practices.

So, while some dismiss the beauty industry as a waste of time and money, it's clear that it serves a deeper purpose. Taking steps to look and feel our best reflects and supports our fundamental need for connection, acceptance and, ultimately, happiness. Or, more simply put, we're worth it.

# PART ONE

## It starts at home

There's no arguing that high-tech treatments can work wonders on our skin. In some instances, they can even reverse damage done by less than diligent skincare practices, such as the ill-advised sunbed habit I developed in my twenties.

That doesn't mean we should put our skin through the wringer, however. If you want the best results, it's important to focus on what I like to call 'pre-juvination'.

This means proactively looking after skin before signs of ageing appear. In my experience, clients who commit to this approach – wherever they are in their ageing journey – see the best outcomes and can even reduce the need for more intensive interventions, such as fillers, as they age.

In this section, I'll explain the science of skin ageing (how and why it occurs) and outline the at-home habits that can stimulate collagen, support skin health and keep you looking and feeling your very best for the long haul.

# Think yourself younger

Looking and feeling our best starts with the way we think. It can be tempting to skip ahead to injectables and quick-fix skin treatments but there's power in laying strong foundations first. Here's why cultivating a positive mindset can make all the difference.

## Our faces reflect our minds

Think of someone you know who always seems to be in a bad mood. Is this reflected in their face? Negative thoughts create facial expressions that, over time, can age us beyond our years. If we're always frowning, we might develop deep frown lines, for instance. Similarly, a generally sullen or sulky demeanour can train muscles to pull downwards, resulting in a permanently unhappy or drooping look.

As Roald Dahl rather bluntly puts it in his childhood classic, *The Twits*, "If a person has ugly thoughts, it begins to show on the face. And when that person has ugly thoughts every day, every week, every year, the face gets uglier and uglier until you can hardly bear to look at it."

On the other hand, embracing a positive mindset can support healthy ageing. When we're happy our facial muscles relax, fostering a more youthful and radiant appearance.

## We are what we think

Speak to any neuroscientist and they'll tell you that our thoughts and feelings trigger the release of various chemicals in the body. Negative emotions encourage the production of stress hormones like cortisol, which can accelerate ageing and lead to adverse health outcomes including hypertension and weakened immunity. On the other hand, cultivating positivity can encourage the release of feel-good hormones, which promote overall wellbeing and act as natural pain relievers.

## Positive thoughts motivate action

Research suggests that people with a sunny outlook are more likely to engage in habits that support good wellbeing, such as regular exercise, a balanced diet, and a proper skincare routine. Meanwhile, a negative mindset can lead to unhealthy behaviours, including poor diet and lack of exercise, which result in a higher risk of chronic illness. We can, quite literally, think ourselves to a happier, healthier life.

## Cultivating a positive mindset

While the idea of adopting a sunnier outlook sounds great, how can we actually create and maintain one? In my experience, this starts with a well-designed morning routine.

By starting the day right – blending positive psychology, wellbeing rituals and beauty best practices – we can set the tone for a happy day. I describe my ideal morning routine on the next page.

**HYDRATION RITUAL** (*1 minute*): Before breakfast, I drink a pint of warm water infused with Ancient + Brave's True Hydration powder (which comprises key minerals for rapid rehydration) or, alternatively, a pinch of Himalayan Sea salt. This simple ritual boosts energy levels, enhances mental clarity, hydrates skin, and supports overall health.

**STAIR WALKING** (*3 minutes*): Next, I energise my body by walking up and down the stairs as quickly as I can. If stairs aren't for you, try star jumps, skipping or running on the spot. We can all find time for three minutes of exercise. It helps to get our heart going, improve circulation and awaken both body and mind.

**BODY BRUSHING** (*2 minutes*): Engaging in a few minutes of dry brushing helps stimulate blood flow and exfoliate the skin. Begin from your feet or hands, brushing in an upward motion towards the heart. This refreshing routine not only revitalises your skin but also aids in cellulite reduction and promotes a glowing complexion. I love the 'zingy' sensation it creates that helps to wake me up!

**INVIGORATING SHOWER** (*6 minutes*): Upgrade your morning shower with a therapeutic scent. I love Clarins Tonic Bath & Shower Concentrate which is enriched with stimulating geranium and rosemary. For the final minute, turn the temperature down and brave the cold water for an extra kick of invigoration (it gets easier, I promise!). Follow up with a firming body cream to moisturise and tone skin.

**STRETCHING** (*5 minutes*): Engage in a short stretching routine to release tension, enhance flexibility, and foster a sense of relaxation. Regular stretching can also aid good mobility in your later years. A yoga sun salutation is one of my favourite moves – you can find lots of simple tutorials on YouTube.

**POSITIVE MEDITATION** (*5-10 minutes*): Dedicate time to a guided meditation or mindfulness practice (I use the Insight Timer app), focusing on fostering gratitude and a positive outlook.

**Total time:** 20-25 minutes

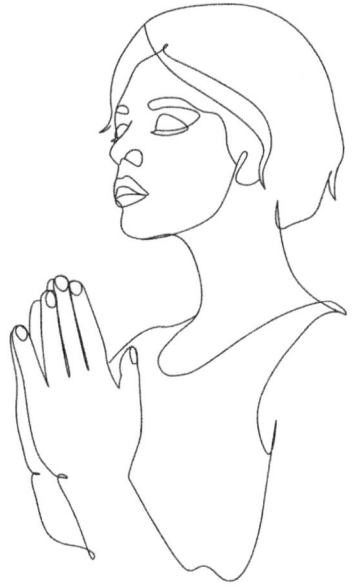

*I promise you that this routine is well worth sacrificing an extra twenty minutes in bed for! While I may not have time to do the entire routine every day, practising just a few of the steps is enough to provide a much-appreciated boost of vitality and positivity.*

# The science of skin ageing

As we journey through life our skin works very hard for us, and so signs of wear and tear are inevitable. Let's take a closer look at the science of ageing so we can better understand how to protect this all-important organ from the inside-out.

## The epidermis – skin cycling

The epidermis has five distinct layers and is our skin's protective outer surface. New skin cells are made in the deepest layer of the epidermis, known as the basal layer. These fresh, juicy skin cells rise up through the layers of the epidermis, maturing as they go. When they reach the skin's surface they naturally shed, making way for new cells. When we're in our 20s, this cycle is super speedy, averaging about 28 days in total. By the time we reach our 60s, things have slowed down quite dramatically – our skin cells can hang around for 50 days or more. The result? A dull, less vibrant complexion.

Our skin cells are likely to look a bit different as we get older too. This is thanks to ultraviolet (UV) rays emitted by the sun which can damage our cell DNA. It is this genetic damage that can lead to the development of blemishes, lesions, sunspots, and other skin abnormalities.

## The dermis – plumping proteins

Below the epidermis is the dermis. This is where proteins such as collagen and elastin – crucial for skin firmness and elasticity – are stored. Picture the dermis as a mattress filled with springs (collagen) and elastic bands (elastin), that provide support and resilience. From our twenties onwards, we lose about one percent of our dermal collagen each year, leading to wrinkles and sagging as the 'mattress' becomes less firm and elastic.

We also find veins in the dermis. As the years pass, these become more visible as the skin thins and the walls of our veins weaken and no longer operate as efficiently. Don't panic – I'll tell you what we can do about all this later.

## The subcutaneous layer – friendly fats

Deeper still is the subcutaneous layer, which is filled with fat that contributes to the skin's plump and youthful look. How much change we're likely to see in the layer depends on our genetics and body weight. You might lose fat, resulting in a hollow appearance, or gain fat, altering the skin's texture and your overall face shape.

## Spare a thought for your skeleton

It's not just our skin that changes as we age: the underlying structures are impacted too.

From midlife onwards, we're likely to lose bone mass, making for a slightly smaller skull (yes, really!). This affects how skin drapes over our facial bones, subtly changing our facial volume and structure. Muscles can also weaken as we age, contributing to a sagging face and body.

Given these complexities, it's clear that a face cream (no matter how pricey or advanced the ingredients) is never going to be able to reverse or halt all the visible signs of ageing. We're going to have to work from the inside-out, drawing on nutrition, exercise and non-surgical treatments too.

# The M word: menopause and your skin

There's no escaping the 'M' word. Yes, I'm talking menopause – a hormonal transition that affects everything from our mood to our sleep, libido and skin. It's not to be underestimated.

Thanks to the hard work of menopause campaigners, and celebs such as Davina McCall, it's finally getting the attention it deserves. In this chapter, I'll explain what menopause means for your skin.

## What is menopause?

The word menopause describes the moment when a woman's periods stop. In fact, medics can officially diagnose menopause when you've not had a period for one year. Yet, most women experience menopause symptoms for a number of months or even years before their periods stop – this time is known as perimenopause.

Symptoms of perimenopause typically start in a woman's mid-to-late forties as the ovaries gradually stop producing eggs and, as a result, levels of hormones called oestrogen, progesterone and testosterone fluctuate and fall.

With our hormones in flux, we may experience mood-related symptoms (such as feeling tense, nervous, anxious, irritable or depressed), as well as physical symptoms such as a racing heartbeat, recurring urinary tract infections, hot flushes, night sweats and muscle and joint pain. What fun!

Many women also report feeling more tired than usual, as well as difficulties with memory, concentration and low libido. It's important to keep in mind that every woman's experience is different. Some will be debilitated by symptoms while others sail through this hormonal change with few adverse effects.

## Menopause and your skin

Every area of a woman's body is affected by hormonal changes and our skin is no different. Oestrogen is a skin-supportive hormone that helps our complexion maintain moisture, elasticity, collagen production, and overall thickness. As oestrogen levels fall during menopause, our skin becomes thinner, more fragile and prone to bruising and tearing. We're left more vulnerable to dry skin as well as increased wrinkles, fine lines and sagging, as collagen production in our skin 'mattress' takes a nosedive too. This is why we might notice a loss of firmness around the cheeks, jawline and neck in midlife.

But that's not all (sorry). Reduced oestrogen levels can lead to an uneven distribution of melanin, creating areas of hyperpigmentation (dark spots) or hypopigmentation (light spots). Some women also experience increased skin sensitivity or irritation during menopause, manifesting as redness, itching, or a burning sensation.

## Can HRT help?

Hormone replacement therapy (also known as HRT) is a medical treatment used to treat menopause symptoms by replenishing levels of oestrogen, progesterone and, in some women, testosterone. It can be prescribed by a GP and comes in various forms including tablets, gels, patches and sprays.

Its primary purpose is to treat symptoms such as night sweats, mood swings, insomnia and vaginal dryness, but there's evidence that replacing hormones can benefit our long-term health too. Research suggests HRT can help to keep bones strong and reduce our risk of osteoporosis, fractures and falls as we age. There's also evidence that HRT can reduce our risk of developing coronary heart disease, or of having a heart attack or stroke.

HRT offers benefits for skin, too. Studies show that 17-β-oestradiol (the body-identical oestrogen prescribed by NHS doctors) can improve skin hydration, reduce wrinkle depth, and enhance collagen production. Therefore, taking HRT may provide some benefits in our quest to maintain smooth, firm, and youthful-looking skin.

For me, hormone therapy has been transformational. I vividly remember the onset of perimenopause although, at the time, I had no idea what was causing my symptoms. Driving on the motorway (a task I had always found routine) suddenly filled me with anxiety. I became overly sensitive to comments and often felt overwhelmed. Running my clinic, a source of pride, began to feel like an insurmountable challenge, and I seriously contemplated closing the business I'd worked so hard to build. Sleep became a challenge too: I used to enjoy settling into bed after a long day, but it was now a source of dread as I fretted about whether I'd spend the night lying awake.

However, just two weeks into HRT therapy, I felt rejuvenated – like a wiser version of my younger self. My symptoms vanished and I don't think I've ever felt as hormonally or psychologically balanced as I do today.

## Is HRT for everyone?

While, for many women, HRT is safe and effective, it's not for everyone. I know women who prefer not to take it and others (such as those with a history of oestrogen-receptive breast cancer) for whom the risks outweigh the benefits.

If you're not sure whether HRT is right for you, I'd recommend speaking with a specialist menopause doctor who can help guide you through the benefits and risks and, if you choose to proceed, tailor the therapy to your specific health profile.

# The gut-skin connection

Gut health is all the rage these days and for good reason. This formerly under-appreciated organ plays a role in everything from the strength of our immune system to our mood and even how well we age.

I've learnt how important it is to take care of our gut (and the microbes that live there) the hard way. Not long ago, I started experiencing indigestion every day, as well as an overwhelming feeling of tiredness. This continued for almost three months before I decided enough was enough – it was time to reach out for help.

I spoke to a registered dietician and attended a week-long gut health retreat. The gut-healthy habits I learned (and will share with you) disappeared my symptoms and I'm pleased to report that I'm now feeling healthy, happy and energised once again.

I didn't expect my gut-friendly habits to have an impact on my appearance, but the results were quite astonishing – I lost weight and saw visible improvements in my skin as the weeks passed. I've since learned that I'm not a one-off. There's a growing body of research suggesting a strong association between a healthy gut and healthy skin. Let's dive in.

## What do we mean by a healthy gut?

A healthy gut is typically characterised by a diverse gut microbiome. This means that the gastrointestinal tract hosts a wide range of microbial species, including bacteria, fungi, viruses, and protozoa. Diversity is crucial, because different microbes perform different functions that contribute to aspects of overall health – including digestion, immunity, and hormone production.

Today, scientists refer to the gut as 'the second brain', due to its role in multiple bodily functions and processes. Some of the main ones include:

### Inflammation

The gut is a key player in regulating inflammation throughout the body. Imbalanced gut bacteria can lead to chronic low-grade inflammation, which is associated with accelerated ageing and skin conditions including eczema, psoriasis, and acne.

### Nutrient absorption

A happy and healthy gut microbiome is vital for optimal nutrient absorption, including vitamins, minerals, and antioxidants that support skin health. Poor gut health can impair nutrient absorption, leading to deficiencies that may contribute to skin ageing and skin disorders.

### Skin barrier function

A balanced gut microbiome helps maintain the integrity of the skin barrier which, when compromised, can lead to increased sensitivity, dryness, and inflammation.

### Hormonal balance

The gut microbiome influences hormone metabolism and signalling pathways, including those involved in skin health. Hormonal imbalances can exacerbate skin concerns and accelerate skin ageing (learn more about this on p 27).

The gut has also been shown to influence the production of serotonin (the 'happy hormone').

# Steps for a happy and healthier gut

Enhancing your gut health doesn't need to be complicated.
Try these simple gut-friendly tweaks.

### Increase your fibre intake

Eat a diverse range of fibre-rich foods, including fruits, vegetables, nuts, seeds, and legumes, to nourish beneficial gut bacteria. Experts now recommend eating about 30 different plant foods a week.
(Don't worry, it doesn't have to be large quantities – herbs and spices count too!) Slow and steady wins the race here. It's wise to very gradually increase your fibre intake to avoid digestive discomfort.

### Go fermented

Aim to add probiotic-rich fermented foods into your diet – such as plain yoghurt, kefir, sauerkraut, and kimchi. These contain 'live' bacteria that can help to supercharge healthy gut activity. Taking a probiotic supplement that is specially formulated for skin health may also be helpful.

### Minimise processed foods

Processed foods, often packed with refined sugars and artificial additives, can disrupt the gut microbiota balance. Avoid processed white carbs like rice, bread, and pasta, and instead focus on obtaining carbs from non-starchy vegetables such as beetroot, celeriac, and swede.

### Try a Mediterranean diet

We frequently hear the Mediterranean diet lauded by experts. One key reason? Research shows that eating a diet packed with plenty of different fruits, vegetables, wholegrains, nuts, and extra virgin olive oil can increase gut bacteria diversity and promote the growth of beneficial bacteria.

**Eat foods rich in polyphenols**

Polyphenols are plant chemicals that give fruits and veggies their bright colours. These colourful chemicals can aid in keeping our gut bacteria balanced by promoting the good guys and supressing the harmful species. Polyphenols are found in lots of different foods, including green tea, berries, red wine (in moderation!), and dark chocolate (skip the milk chocolate that's high in sugar and can negatively impact the gut microbiome).

**Reduce your alcohol intake**

I'm not saying you should never enjoy the odd tipple. But excessive alcohol consumption can harm the gut microbiome by promoting inflammation and reducing the diversity of beneficial bacteria. Learn more about the impact alcohol has on skin on p.40.

**Manage stress**

Research suggests our gut hates stress just as much as we do. Excessive stress levels can cause digestive issues such as bloating, constipation, diarrhoea and stomach aches. Studies also show that stress can disrupt skin barrier function and worsen inflammatory conditions such as eczema, acne and psoriasis.

I know that keeping stress under control is easier said than done! However, relaxation techniques (such as deep breathing), a mindfulness practice, regular exercise and sufficient sleep can work wonders.

Stick with these approaches for a few months and you will reap the rewards – including a clearer, healthier and glowing complexion. If you have a specific gut-related concern or skin condition, be sure to consult with a medical profession or registered dietician for personalised recommendations.

# Am I drinking enough water?

Two is the magic number of litres it's recommended we drink each day to maintain good hydration and keep our bodies functioning at their best. But do these benefits extend to our skin as well? Drum roll... yes! Let's take a closer look at the evidence.

**Improved skin hydration**
Research shows that drinking plenty of water can positively impact skin hydration levels. For instance, one study found that drinking two or more litres of water per day improved both superficial and deep skin hydration – particularly among those who had previously drunk less water.

**Improved skin elasticity and reduced wrinkles**
Studies indicate that drinking enough water can improve skin elasticity and reduce wrinkle depth. When skin is better hydrated at the cellular level, its stronger, smoother and more resilient.

**Enhanced skin barrier function**
There's also evidence that keeping hydrated can support our skin's barrier function. If its barrier remains strong, skin leaks less moisture throughout the day and is better protected against the environmental stressors that contribute to ageing.

# Working up a thirst for better skin

**If you're anything like me, drinking two litres of water a day can pose a challenge. Here are the strategies I put in place to take me from H²-no to H²-go:**

1. Purchase a water bottle that's marked with hourly reminders. This will motivate you to drink regularly.

2. Carry a water bottle with you wherever you go – whether at work, in the car, or at the gym.

3. Infuse water with slices of fruit, such as lemon or cucumber (yep, cucumber is technically a fruit, not a veggie). Adding natural flavours can make water more enjoyable to drink.

4. Drink a glass of water ten minutes before each meal. This is known as habit stacking – linking a new habit with another activity we already perform regularly. I've noticed this burst of hydration also helps me feel full more quickly, making portion control easier.

5. Eat lots of water-rich foods such as watermelon, cucumber, and oranges. The water in these foods contribute to our overall hydration levels.

## What about tea and coffee?

Around three-quarters of adults start their day with a cup of java. But what impact does this have on skin?

As caffeine is known to have a diuretic effect (meaning it can increase urine production), some worry that their morning coffee might lead to dehydration. However, research reveals that moderate coffee consumption is unlikely to cause significant dehydration. While high levels of caffeine can increase urine output, the effect is relatively mild, especially in regular coffee drinkers. The key to avoiding any potential dehydration from coffee (and the knock-on effects on skin) is to ensure you drink plenty of water throughout the day.

So, enjoying your morning coffee is unlikely to harm your skin health, as long as it's long as it's paired with plenty of water too. And that caffeine kick first thing may even provide a few skin-friendly antioxidant benefits!

# Sweet talk: the truth about sugar

Sadly, there's nothing very sweet about this: evidence strongly suggests that consuming excessive amounts of sugar is terrible for our skin.

There are several ways that a sweet tooth can harm efforts to age well.

### Advanced glycation end products (AGEs)

When sugar molecules in the bloodstream bind to proteins, they form harmful compounds known as AGE. AGEs can damage collagen and elastin, contributing to wrinkles and sagging skin.

### Inflammation

When we eat lots of sugar, we trigger inflammation in the body, leading to oxidative stress and cell damage. Chronic inflammation accelerates the ageing process and is associated with various skin conditions, including acne, eczema, and psoriasis.

### Collagen degradation

Eating too much sugar can disrupt the structure and function of collagen fibres in skin. When collagen becomes damaged or degraded, the skin may appear dull, wrinkled, and aged.

Thus, reducing your sugar intake can help you age well inside and out.

# Here are my tips for keeping a sweet tooth under control

**Start the day right**

If we can swerve sugary foods first-thing, and keep our blood sugar levels balanced, we're more likely to stay on track for the rest of the day. This is because blood sugar spikes (and the crash that follows) can contribute to the mid-afternoon sugar cravings that find us reaching for a biscuit. My first meal tends to consist of protein-rich foods such as eggs or yoghurt for a more balanced start to the day.

**Go to the dark side**

If chocolate is your weakness, try to opt for darker varieties which are lower in sugar and packed full of skin-friendly antioxidants. If your tastebuds have grown used to super-sweet milk or white chocolate, start with a lower 60-70% cocoa percentage to begin with, before slowly working your way up to darker varieties. Get creative with flavours, too. My favourite dark chocolate bars are infused with sweet cherry, spicy chilli and zesty lime.

**Pass on pop**

When trying to limit sugar, ditching sugary drinks is the easiest place to start. Swap these empty calories with flavoured water or even gut-friendly kombucha (a delicious, fermented tea that populates the gut with skin-healthy microbes). I steer clear of 'sugar-free' drinks that are loaded with artificial sweeteners – these can also spike our blood sugar.

# You booze, you lose

Research shows younger generations are drinking less alcohol than ever before, but us older folk aren't making the same shifts. In fact, midlife women are particularly guilty of over-indulging: figures show that we're most likely to exceed recommended drinking limits between the age of 45 to 64, with almost one in five (19%) of us drinking more than 14 units of alcohol a week.

We know that too much booze can compromise our health and increase our risk of chronic disease, but it's also bad news for our skin. If you're on the fence about whether to reduce your alcohol intake, I'm hoping these skin facts will give you the final push:

**Dehydration**
As a diuretic, alcohol makes us need the toilet more frequently which can lead to dehydration – particularly if we're not remembering to order a glass of water with every alcoholic drink. When we're chronically dehydrated, skin looks dull, dry, and less elastic, making fine lines and wrinkles more noticeable.

**Inflammation**
Drinking alcohol can trigger inflammation in the body, making skin conditions such as acne, rosacea, and eczema worse. If levels of inflammation remain high (known as chronic inflammation) this can also accelerate the ageing process and contribute to the breakdown of skin-plumping collagen and elastin.

**Skin redness**

Have you ever noticed your cheeks turning pink as you drink? This happens because alcohol encourages our blood vessels to relax. This increases blood flow to the face, making skin appear red and feel warm to the touch. This is particularly noticeable in those who have rosacea, a skin concern characterised by facial redness and flushing.

**Puffiness and swelling**

Excessive alcohol intake can cause fluid retention, leading to puffiness in the face and under-eye area and creating a tired appearance.

**Diet disruptor**

Alcohol interferes with the body's ability to absorb and make use of essential nutrients that are crucial for skin health. In other words, it gets in the way of our body getting all the goodness it needs from the food we eat. Over time, this can lead to nutrient deficiencies which contribute to skin dullness and dryness, as well as hair loss and accelerated ageing.

## How to tone down your tipple

*If you find the thought of cutting back on alcohol daunting, here are a few strategies that might help.*

**Create a reward system**

Remember the star charts you created for your kids, or perhaps still make for your grandkids? Switch things up a gear and create your own adult-friendly reward system. Set yourself personal targets for alcohol-free periods – this could be a week, a month, or even six months – and plan meaningful rewards to celebrate these milestones. It might be a meal out, night away or perhaps even one of the skin-rejuvenating treatments described in this book.

**Link alcohol reduction to personal goals**
What do you most want to achieve in this chapter of your life and could drinking a little less help you along the way? When we make a direct connection between (often not so fun) healthy habits and our goals, it's easier to stay motivated when the going gets tough.

For instance, if you're hoping to improve your health and lose some weight, you might remind yourself of this goal when you find yourself tempted to order a glass of wine. Similarly, if you have a professional goal – and know you need a clear head and plenty of energy to pull it off – let this be the motivation you need to swerve a hangover and get yourself to bed early.

# The midlife hangover

I can't bear the 'morning after' feeling nowadays. As I've gotten older, I'm much more likely to wake up with a hangover and my symptoms are more severe too. Sometimes even just a couple of glasses of wine are enough to leave me feeling tired, headachy and sub-par the next day, while my partner escapes unscathed. The culprit? Menopause.

As we enter menopause, hormonal changes can affect our body's ability to break down alcohol and lead to more pronounced hangovers. One key factor is the decline in a liver enzyme called alcohol dehydrogenase (ADH). Women generally produce less ADH than men, but levels can sink even further after menopause, resulting in higher blood alcohol levels after just a few drinks and more severe hangover symptoms.

Research also shows that a woman's liver can shrink by up to 40% during perimenopause, which further limits how well we can tolerate alcohol.

All the more reason to make sure we're pairing our alcoholic drinks with water and that we're mindful of our intake from midlife onwards.

# Why am I ageing faster than my friends?

The ageing process doesn't follow a predictable timeline and, contrary to what scarily convincing Instagram filters will have you believe, it's impossible to predict how you'll look in 20 years' time.

We all age on a unique schedule, set for us by our genetics and lifestyle habits. Here's what we can and can't control.

## What you can't control

Intrinsic ageing describes skin changes driven by the genetic hand we've been dealt. Just as we inherit our eye colour or height from our parents, we also inherit traits that determine how our skin will age – such as skin colour. Fair-skinned individuals (especially redheads and light blondes) tend to age more quickly. They have lower levels of protective pigment in their skin, which unfortunately makes them more susceptible to sunburn and premature ageing.

We also carry genetic variations that affect our skin's elasticity, hydration, and antioxidant defences – key factors that influence how quickly we're likely to show signs of ageing. For instance, certain genetic markers can make some people more prone to wrinkles, skin laxity, or dry skin.

Sadly, we can't edit our ageing genes any more than we can will our eyes to change colour. The good news, however, is that intrinsic factors account for just 20% of the ageing process. That leaves 80% firmly within our control.

## What you can control

Extrinsic ageing describes the skin changes triggered by our environment. This includes how diligently we apply sun protection, our exposure to pollution and our lifestyle choices – such as the quality of our diet and whether or not we smoke.

Take my grandparents, for example. My late grandmother, a chronic worrier with a deep affection for Cadbury's milk chocolate, was a light but regular smoker her entire life – as were many women of her generation. She developed deep lines and wrinkles early in life. In contrast, my grandfather – a quiet, mild-mannered man who quit smoking early and rarely indulged in sweets – maintained a smooth, almost wrinkle-free complexion well into his later years. Coincidence? I think not.

Add to that a new field of science known as epigenetics and we may well have more control over our speed of ageing than we think. We can't change our genes, but research now shows we can influence how these genes express themselves, with our lifestyle choices exaggerating or minimising their effects. The healthy habits that can limit less favourable genes include all the usual suspects: adopting a healthy diet, managing stress, getting adequate sleep, avoiding smoking, using effective skincare treatments and protecting skin from sunlight.

I can't stress the importance of sun protection enough. This is the number one cause of accelerated skin ageing I see in the clinic – showing up as damaged elastin and collagen fibres, skin wrinkles, age spots and sagging skin. Your future is in your hands.

# Smart skincare

Have you ever tried a cream on the back of your hand in store, noticed an immediate improvement and decided to buy it – only to later be disappointed by the lack of long-term results? Yup, me too. It's frustrating, especially when we've splashed the cash. Here's what's likely going on in these instances.

As I explained earlier, the outermost layer of skin is made of old, dry skin cells. When you apply a moisturising cream to this layer, it hydrates the dead cells leaving skin looking temporarily plump and radiant. *Temporarily* is the key word here. The results quickly fade once surface-level swelling and shine evaporates away.

For products to have a longer lasting, meaningful impact they need to work their way into the deeper structures of our skin. This means prioritising quality over quantity when it comes to skincare and hunting down the evidence-based technologies that deliver real results.

## Read the label

As we've established, not all skincare products are created equal. Always read the label and take time to look at the ingredients you're spending your money on. The very best ingredients penetrate the deeper layers of skin and have been shown to deliver visible improvements in clinical trials. Here are the key players to look out for.

## Peptides

Peptides stimulate collagen production and tighten skin, resulting in a firmer appearance.

## Vitamin C

This powerful antioxidant slows down the ageing process by fighting oxidative stress caused by sun damage and pollution. Vitamin C can also help to brighten the complexion and supports collagen production.

## Niacinamide

Known for its anti-inflammatory properties, niacinamide is effective in treating rosacea, acne, and other inflammatory skin conditions.

## Green tea

Rich in antioxidants, green tea helps combat acne and has anti-ageing benefits due to its ability to fight free-radical damage.

## Exfoliating acids

Exfolliating acids such as lactic, malic and fruit acids work by breaking the bonds between dead skin cells, promoting cell turnover for fresher, younger-looking skin. They are often more effective exfoliants than traditional face scrubs and can be found in liquid toners, serums, or masks.

## Tyrosinase inhibitors

If you're struggling with skin pigmentation, it's well worth hunting down this family of skin ingredients as they block the formation of melanin – the pigment in skin that contributes to dark spots, sun damage and melasma. My favourites include liquorice and arbutin.

## Hyaluronic acid

A hydrating powerhouse, hyaluronic acid replenishes skin's moisture leaving it supple and plump.

**Sunscreen**

Don't skip this essential pro-ageing ingredient. Sunscreen is key for protecting the skin from harmful UV rays, reducing skin cancer risk and preventing premature ageing.

The two types of rays that pose a threat to our skin are UVA and UVB rays (we're protected from UVC rays by the ozone layer). That's why it's important to look for sunscreens that offer broad-spectrum protection against both.

There are two types of sunscreens – chemical and physical.

Chemical sunscreens contain carbon-derived ingredients, such as oxybenzone. They work by creating a chemical reaction that changes UV rays into heat, and this heat is then released from the skin. By absorbing UV radiation before it penetrates the skin, these sunscreens prevent damage from occurring in deeper layers.

Chemical sunscreens typically feel lighter on the skin and don't leave any streaky white traces associated with the sunscreens of old. They usually need to be applied about 30 minutes before you go outside for maximum efficacy and are ideal for holidays as they do not come off as easily when we sweat.

Physical sunscreens contain mineral ingredients such as titanium dioxide or zinc oxide. They sit on the surface of skin and physically block and scatter UV rays (think of them like a medieval knight's shield on your arm).

These sunscreens are often thicker and may leave a white cast on the skin. While less aesthetically pleasing, this cast provides a visible assurance of coverage. You can avoid this by opting for less visible, micronised zinc oxide.

**Retinol**

This ingredient isn't a skincare buzzword for nothing. A derivative of vitamin A, retinol encourages the growth of new cells and exfoliates the skin from the inside-out, speeding up cell turnover and collagen production for reduced wrinkles and improved skin texture. It's the gold-standard anti-ageing ingredient with years of research to back up its claims.

## A NOTE ON RETINOL

While retinol's benefits are certainly appealing, it's important to take things slow if you're a vitamin A newbie. First, patch test the product to check for an adverse reaction. If all is well, you can then begin with a low percentage dose, gradually increasing the number of times you apply the serum over a period of weeks and months. For example, I tend to recommend that clients start by applying retinol just twice a week, before increasing it to three times a week after fourteen days or so. From there, you can continue to increase the dose until you're using your retinol most evenings. You can even up the percentage once your skin has fully acclimatised.

If you find that your skin feels tight or red after retinol use, take a break until skin returns to normal. This is known as a 'retinol response' and can be avoided by applying a moisturiser directly after your retinol.

You're also more likely to experience sensitivity if the retinol you're applying doesn't have a well-designed delivery system. For this reason, I always recommend buying a retinoid from your local MediSpa, rather than online. Most MediSpas (including my own) offer high-quality cosmeceutical skincare lines, which undergo rigorous testing to ensure they're safe and effective. A good clinic will also offer complimentary consultations, during which a skincare professional will recommend products according to your specific skin concerns, such as ageing, pigmentation, acne, rosacea, and dehydration.

## Your skincare routine

When it comes to skincare, consistency is key. You can't apply a serum and expect to see overnight results. But, if you diligently apply quality products (day and night) you will see improvements in skin texture, tone and resilience, as well as a reduction in fine lines, redness and pigmentation.

Beware of switching out products too regularly. When carrying out skin consultations at my MediSpa clinic, I often discover clients are following what I call a 'mishmash' routine – subscribing to skincare clubs which post out surprise products each month. While this might be good fun, it's not going to deliver age-defying results.

### Be brand loyal

If you want the best results, pick one skincare brand – preferably a cosmeceutical range from your local MediSpa – and don't use anything else. This ensures products have been designed to work together and takes all the guesswork out of layering and combining the products. My favourite cosmeceutical brands include Alumier MD (I use this), as well as Skinceuticals, ZO Skin Health and mesoestetic.

## Morning routine

A well-designed morning routine brightens and hydrates the skin for a radiant and wide-awake look, while also protecting against any UV or environmental damage we might encounter throughout the day. As you can see, it doesn't need to be a complicated routine. By investing in a few high-quality products, we can set our skin up for success.

**1. Cleanser:** Cleanse skin thoroughly to remove makeup and dirt, and prepare your skin for the next steps.

**2. Toner:** Most cosmeceutical skincare ranges come with a pH-balanced cleanser, in which case a toner is not required. If not, a gentle acid toner can help restore skin acidity.

**3. Serums:** The powerhouse in your skincare routine, serums deliver the biggest concentration of the pro-ageing ingredients listed above. Choose a serum that addresses your biggest skin concern, whether that be hyperpigmentation, ageing or something else altogether. I recommend looking for multi-ingredient serums that contain vitamin C to protect against oxidative stress; hyaluronic acid to hydrate skin and support barrier function; and peptides to stimulate collagen and firm the skin.

**4. Eye cream:** Gently pat a small amount of eye cream around the orbital bone and below the brow bone to hydrate and protect the delicate skin around the eyes. Your morning eye cream should contain skin brightening ingredients, such as vitamin C to tackle dark circles, and peptides to boost collagen production. Niacinamide and hyaluronic acid can also help to plump and hydrate skin.

**5. SPF moisturiser:** Most cosmeceutical ranges combine a moisituriser and physical sunscreen into one convenient product. If your moisturiser does not contain SPF, be sure to apply a separate broad-spectrum sunscreen as your final skincare step.

**6. Primer:** If desired, apply a primer after sunscreen to blur pores and fine lines, creating a smooth canvas for makeup application. My favourite is the Alumier Vitamin Rich Smoother, but I also like Charlotte Tilbury's primers.

## Evening routine

While we sleep, our skin is busy at work repairing damaged cells and rebuilding skin-plumping collagen. The best evening skincare routines supply our skin with everything it needs to do this job to its best ability.

**1. Cleanser:** Begin your night-time routine by thoroughly cleansing your skin to remove makeup, dirt, and excess oil.

**2. Serum:** I'd recommend a powerful serum that contains pro-ageing ingredients such as retinol and peptides. Keep this away from the delicate skin around the eyes.

**3. Eye cream:** Again, retinol and peptides are the key ingredients to prioritise but in a gentler, more nourishing formula that's better suited to thin skin around the eyes.

**4. Night cream:** Finish with a moisturiser that contains ingredients such as peptides, niacinamide, green tea, vitamin E and hyaluronic acid to replenish moisture, support skin regeneration and protect against damaging free radicals.

## Helpful extras

**Exfoliators:** If skin is looking dull or uneven in texture, reach for an exfoliating acid. Use these 2-3 times a week to speed up cell turnover and keep skin looking its best. Lactic acid is a great option for ageing skin as it's hydrating and calming.

**Masks:** These are very relaxing to apply and are a great way of introducing some fun (and any new ingredients you'd like to try) into your skincare practices, without disrupting your tried-and-tested routine.

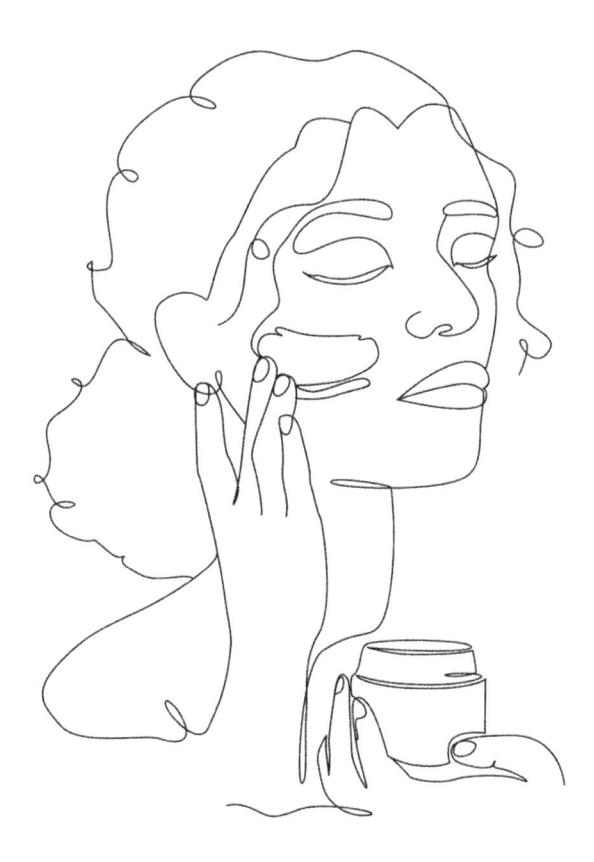

# Beauty sleep

We know that sleep is crucial for overall health and our skin is no different – they don't call it beauty sleep for nothing!

However, not all slumber is good for our looks. I've seen many clients unwittingly sabotage their skincare efforts overnight, quite literally pressing deep wrinkles (known as sleep creases) into their face with their pillow.

## What causes sleep creases?

Sleep creases are wrinkles that form due to the repeated pressure and folding of the skin during sleep, particularly if we tend to sleep on our sides or stomach.

These creases can appear on our face but also on the decolletage – particularly if we sleep on our sides. This is because the skin between breasts is repeatedly compressed in this position.

Our sleeping position becomes more important as we age as the loss of collagen and elastin reduces skin's natural ability to bounce back. The creases formed during sleep take longer to disappear and can eventually become permanently etched into the skin.

# Keep skin smooth while sleeping

**Here's everything you need to know to emerge from a great night's sleep with your skin unscathed**

### Back sleeping
The most effective way to prevent sleep creases is to lie on your back at night. This position avoids putting pressure on the face and décolletage, allowing the skin to remain smooth throughout the night. However, changing sleep positions can be challenging, especially for those (like me) who naturally prefer to sleep on their sides.

I have that found that placing a pillow under my knees when lying on my back can help maintain a comfortable position and reduce the tendency to turn onto my side.

### Try a face pillow
For committed side sleepers, uniquely designed pillows such as the Face Pillow can be a game-changer. Available online, these support the head in a way that reduces pressure on the face and encourages back sleeping.

Be patient and persistent – adjusting to a new sleep position or using a special pillow can take time. Trust that your body will adapt, and your skin will thank you.

# PART TWO

## Find your fix

Now that we've nailed a 'pre-juvenation' approach to taking care of our skin, we can move on to more targeted treatments. Clients come to my MediSpa with a wide range of concerns – from hyperpigmentation and under-eye circles to droopy jowls, frown lines and turkey neck. I've seen it all over the years!

If there's a particular 'problem area' that's chipping away at your self-esteem, rest assured there's always something that can be done. In the following pages, I'll explore the most common aesthetic concerns, why they occur and how (in my experience) they're best treated.

For more detailed information on the treatments and technologies mentioned, please refer to the treatment index (p126).

# Turkey neck

Turkey neck is the apt (albeit unpleasant) name given to sagging skin that can appear between our chin and neck as we age.

## What causes turkey neck?

Skin strength, muscle tone and fat distribution can all play a role in how wobbly our under-chin area appears. Here's what you need to know.

**Mind your muscles**
You know where to find your biceps, but have you heard of the digastric muscle? This teeny muscle is found under the jaw and can become more prominent as we age, creating an undesirable bulge. And, like the muscles in our arms or legs, the digastric muscle can lose tone and elasticity as we get older, creating a saggy appearance.

Meanwhile, the platysma muscle (which lies over the diagastric muscle) also becomes lax with age. This creates vertical bands across the neck which contribute to that wobbly turkey neck look.

**Fat chance**
If fat deposits build up under our chin (known to those in aesthetics as submentum fat accumulation), the neck can develop a saggy and bulging appearance. This excess fat can also push skin and

underlying muscles downward, making matters worse. This is more likely to occur if we're overweight, but our genes play a role too. You can learn more about how to treat a 'double chin' on p.71.

**Protein power**
As you'll have gathered by now, collagen and elastin help to keep skin tight and toned. As levels of these proteins naturally decline with age, the result is increased sagging and wrinkling – particularly in the delicate neck area.

## Treatments for turkey neck

The good news is there's plenty we can do – both at-home and in-clinic – to tighten and tone a turkey neck.

## For reversing muscle changes:

### HIFES
HIFES or high-intensity electromagnetic stimulation is a workout for the face, helping to strengthen and tighten the digastric and platysma muscles that run from the chin to the neck. The result? You can wave your wobble goodbye.

### Toxin injections
Not just for banishing wrinkles, toxin injections (better known by the brand name – Botox) can temporarily relax the troublesome muscles that pull skin downwards, resulting in a smoother neck. These are particularly useful when it comes to softening vertical neck bands.

## For tackling under chin fat:

### Synchronised radiofrequency
There are various ways to tackle fat under the chin but, in my opinion, this is the safest and most effective. The special technology reaches a hotter temperature than you'd see in standard radiofrequency treatments. This heat melts away unwanted fat cells and improves the contour of the neck.

### Other fat-busters
Some clinics offer cryolipolysis – a 'fat freezing' approach that eliminates stubborn fat cells with icy temperatures. You may also find lipolysis injections at your local MediSpa. These contain deoxycholic acid which works to dissolve unwanted fat cells. Read more about the pros and cons of these treatments on p.160.

## For lifting and tightening skin:

### Sofwave™
This evidence-based, ultrasound treatment has secured FDA-approval for the treatment of turkey neck. It lifts and tightens the neck and submentum (under chin) area with targeted parallel beam technology that stimulates collagen, elastin and hyaluronic acid. This leads to smoother, firmer-looking skin and a more defined jawline and neck.

### Energy devices
Technologies such as radiofrequency, laser therapy and ultrasound can be used to heat the deeper layers of skin, triggering increased collagen and elastin production for a more contoured neck and chin.

**Skin-boosting injections**

Like a skin serum on steroids, these regenerative injectables deliver hyaluronic acid, peptides, or polynucleotides into the deeper layers of skin where they can stimulate collagen and elastin production. The result? Improved skin quality and firmness.

---

## Try this at home

- Skincare ingredients, such as peptides and retinoids, can help improve skin firmness and texture by promoting collagen production and skin cell turnover.

- Be mindful of your posture. Constantly looking down at our digital devices is wreaking havoc with our necks – a phenomenon now known as 'tech neck'. Try to keep your head upright when using your phone or reduce screen time.

# Frown lines

Frown (or glabellar) lines are the vertical wrinkles that appear between our eyebrows as we age. Read on to discover why these lines appear, as well as the non-surgical treatments that can iron them out.

## What causes frown lines?

Remember what we learned about positive thinking in Part One? Our mood, mindset and facial expressions all play a role in how we look, and frown lines are a prime example.

**Turn that frown upside down**
It's in the name – frown lines are caused by frowning. When we furrow our brow, we make use of muscles in the glabellar region. If we repeatedly contract these muscles over days, weeks, months and years, we create permanent lines in the skin.

**Sands of time**
Ageing (yup, that old chestnut) affects our skin's elasticity and how well it can recover from being folded. Just as our knees and joints can feel creakier in later life, the same is true of our skin – it's less able to bounce back, and so wrinkles are more likely to appear.

## Treatments for frown lines

In my experience, there's only one treatment that will make a significant difference to frown lines and that's Botox. Collagen-stimulating treatments alone are unlikely to produce significant results because the muscles involved in frowning are so strong.

**Toxin injections**

Toxin injections (better known by the brand name – Botox) are the most effective treatment for frown lines and can also act as a good preventative. They temporarily relax the muscles that fold skin and create wrinkles.

### A NOTE ON BOTOX

Be sure to choose a well-trained practitioner as, in the wrong hands, this treatment can result in a brow lift and permanently surprised expression. The key is adding a small injection of toxin higher up on the forehead to mitigate this unwanted effect.

**Energy devices**

Following toxin injections, treatments such as radiofrequency, fractional radiofrequency, ultrasound, Sofwave™, and laser can help stimulate collagen production. This restores bounce to skin and can further soften frown lines.

## Try this at home

- While not as effective as injectables, wearing stick-on anti-frown patches (such as from *frownies.co.uk*) can help to prevent overnight frowning and smooth lines.

- Practising meditation and deep breathing can encourage a calmer mood and reduce frowning frequency.

# Nose-to-mouth lines

Nose-to-mouth lines, aka 'smile lines' or nasolabial folds (to use the clinical term), are the creases that run from the bottom corners of your nose to the corners of your mouth. They are a perfectly natural feature but can become more prominent as we get older.

## What causes nose-to-mouth lines?

As we discovered in Part One, our skin, facial fat, muscles and bones change as we age. This constant evolution can make developing defined smile lines more likely.

**What goes up...**
...must come down (unfortunately). We may have hated our chubby cheeks in early life, but facial fat actually contributes to a youthful look. As we get older, however, this fat slowly disappears and can also drift downwards. The result? Lines become more noticeable.

**Final stretch**
Collagen and elastin production slows as we age, leaving us with thinner, less elastic skin that is more prone to sagging and wrinkling.

**Express yourself**

While I'm not suggesting we aim to never move our mouths, repeated contraction of facial muscles (such as when we smile, laugh, or talk) can gradually etch lines into the face.

## Treatments for nose-to-mouth lines

The best treatments for smile lines work to lift skin and restore lost volume. Here's what I'd recommend.

**Filler**

If lines are very deep, subtle and accurately placed filler is often the best option.

**Sofwave™**

With its unique parallel beam delivery mechanism, Sofwave™ can significantly lift the skin and reduce nose-to-mouth lines.

**HIFES**

HIFES (or high intensity facial electromagnetic stimulation) can help to lift and build cheek muscles, softening nose-to-mouth lines in the process.

**Energy devices**

Radiofrequency, ultrasound and laser treatments can help to stimulate collagen production. Over time, this can help to soften lines.

**Skin-boosting injections**

Skin-boosting injections containing hyaluronic acid, peptides or polynucleotides can help to stimulate collagen production and soften smile lines.

## Try this at home

- While skincare alone is unlikely to erase existing smile lines, daily use of a broad-spectrum SPF can help to slow skin ageing.

- Invest in a good quality (preferably cosmeceutical) retinol or peptide serum. This will help to smooth and plump skin.

- Try sleeping on your back and investing in a silk pillowcase.

# Marionette lines

Marionette lines are the vertical creases or folds that extend from the corners of the mouth down towards the chin. They can create a down-turned, 'sad' expression as they deepen with age.

## What causes marionette lines?

There's no area of the face left untouched by the sands of time – from our skin to our facial fat and muscles. Here's why these changes can contribute to marionette lines:

**Time will tell**

As we age, our skin produces less collagen and elastin, the proteins responsible for keeping skin firm and smooth. This loss of elasticity allows lines and wrinkles to form more easily, particularly in areas of the face that move frequently, like the mouth. UV exposure accelerates this process. If we've spent lots of time in the sun, we're more likely to see a loss of skin structure and resilience. And then there's gravity to contend with. This downward pull can cause skin to sag, creating creases where skin is naturally thinner, such as around the mouth and chin.

## Face off

As with most deeper wrinkles, repetitive facial expressions play a role in the formation of marionette lines. Our facial muscles can also change with age, getting gradually weaker and more elongated. We're also likely to lose facial fat with age – particularly in the mid-face area. This loss of muscle tone and fat leaves skin with less structural support, making sagging and wrinkling more likely.

### Treatments for marionette lines

We can smooth marionette lines by restoring facial volume, relaxing mischievous muscles and lifting sagging skin. Here's what I'd recommend.

**Filler**

If lines are very deep, subtle and accurately placed filler is often the best option. Hyaluronic acid filler is often used for this purpose, delivering immediate but temporary results.

**Sofwave™**

With its unique parallel beam delivery mechanism, Sofwave™ can significantly lift the skin, encourage collagen production and minimise marionette lines.

**Energy devices**

Radiofrequency, ultrasound and laser treatments can help to stimulate collagen production. Over time, this can help to soften lines.

**Toxin injections**

For some people, Botox injections around the corners of the mouth can help to relax the muscles that pull down on the skin. This softens marionette lines.

**Skin-boosting injections**

Skin-boosting injections containing hyaluronic acid, peptides or polynucleotides can help to stimulate collagen production and soften lines.

**Thread lift**

Less invasive than a surgical facelift, thread lifts add structure to sagging skin and minimise lines and creases.

**HIFES**

HIFES (or high intensity facial electromagnetic stimulation) can help to lift and build cheek muscles, softening marionette lines in the process.

---

## Try this at home

- Look for skincare products that contain collagen-boosting ingredients such as retinol and peptides.
- Wear your sunscreen daily.

# Double chin

Ever looked in the mirror to discover you've grown a second chin? You're far from alone as this is one of the most common complaints I see in my clinic. Don't despair, there's plenty that can be done.

## What causes a double chin?

A double chin can appear when a layer of fat accumulates below the jaw. There are a few reasons why this can happen:

**Size matters**

Double chins are often associated with weight gain. But, while it's true that being overweight can contribute to excess fat anywhere on our face, it's perfectly possible to develop a double chin at a healthy weight.

**Keep it in the family**

Genetics plays a significant role in all aspects of our appearance, including where our body likes to store fat. If any close family members (such as a parent or grandparent) have a double chin, we're more likely to develop one.

**Old news**

As we age, a loss of skin firmness can contribute to a double chin. As can age-related changes to where our body chooses to store fat. Excess pounds that may have been more evenly distributed in our youth can start accumulating in unflattering places, including under the chin – what fun!

## Treatments to help reduce a double chin

The only way to treat a double chin is by removing excess fat. But you don't need to go under the knife. Here's how it's done:

### Synchronised radiofrequency

In my experience, this is a safe and effective method for tackling a double chin. The radiofrequency energy creates high temperatures that melt fat cells and improve the contour of the neck.

### Other fat-busters

Some clinics offer cryolipolysis – a 'fat freezing' approach that eliminates stubborn fat cells with icy temperatures. You may also find lipolysis injections at your local MediSpa. These contain deoxycholic acid which dissolves fat cells. Read more about the pros and cons of these treatments on p.160.

## Try this at home

- Taking steps to lose weight can help to reduce the appearance of a double chin. Here's where I'd start:

**1.** Prioritise vegetables, fruit, lean proteins and wholegrains on your plate. These healthy foods promote both fat loss and skin health.

**2.** Avoid processed foods and sugary or salty snacks. These are easy to overeat and can lead to water retention and bloating in the face.

**3.** Stay hydrated. Drinking plenty of water can help to prevent overeating as well as maintain our skin elasticity. It can also help to reduce puffiness.

# Drooping jowls

Remember the cartoon dog, Droopy? He got his name for a reason. Sagging jowls can leave us looking miserable – and, when looking in the mirror, it's hard not to be bothered by them. This is one of the most common concerns I hear from clients, so let's dive into the non-surgical solutions.

## What causes drooping jowls?

As we age, our skin, facial muscles and fat fall victim to gravity, creating a droopy appearance.

**Feel the pull**
As levels of skin-strengthening proteins (collagen and elastin) decline with age, skin can become lax and saggy. Add gravity into the mix and our increasingly fragile faces don't stand a chance. This persistent downward force wins out and we start to see the tell-tale drooping associated with jowls.

**Weakest link**
Muscles in the lower face can weaken over time as a result of genetics, lifestyle factors, and natural ageing processes. This makes jowls more likely to appear.

**On the move**
As we age, we might notice changes to where fat sits on our face

– it might move downwards or start to accumulate in unflattering places. Both can make jowls appear more prominent.

## Bare bones

Our bones are likely to lose density as we get older, and our facial skeleton is no different. A smaller skull can contribute to jowls as there's less support for our facial muscles which then sag.

## Treatments for drooping jowls

Good news: there are plenty of tools we can use to lift and minimise jowls.

### HIFES
High intensity facial electromagnetic stimulation can be used to strengthen and tighten the main cheek muscle. This increases cheek volume and lifts the jowl area – a two-for-one deal! HIFES can also be used to tighten muscles under the chin and down the neck for a more contoured look.

### Sofwave™
Much like HIFES, this innovative, ultrasound treatment can significantly tighten and lift jowls, but this device works on the skin – stimulating collagen, elastin and hyaluronic acid.

### Energy devices
Radiofrequency, ultrasound and laser treatments deliver heat energy into the skin's deeper layers, stimulating collagen production and tightening loose skin. This can help to firm up saggy jowls.

**Toxin injections**
Toxin injections minimise jowls by 'freezing' facial muscles responsible for pulling skin downwards. Strategic injections along the jawline and neck can create a smoother and more lifted silhouette. I've seen brilliant results when toxin injections are combined with Sofwave™ technology.

**Skin-boosting injections**
Injections containing collagen and elastin-stimulating ingredients (think hyaluronic acid, peptides and polynucleotides) can improve skin quality and firmness. This, in turn, can help to tighten and lift the jowl area.

**Filler**
When strategically placed in the cheek area, filler can help to minimise jowls by adding lift and extra support to the mid-face. When applied along the jawline, these injections can also add definition and improve the shape of the lower face.

> **A NOTE ON FILLER**
>
> When it comes to treating jowls with filler, less is more. Be sure to find an experienced and skilled injector, as overfilling the cheeks or jawline can lead to an unnatural or exaggerated look. When done well, filler looks subtle and balanced.

**Facial threads**
Like a push-up bra for the face, threads provide an immediate mechanical lift that can contour the jawline and minimise drooping. This treatment also stimulates collagen production for more resilient and youthful-looking skin.

> ## Try this at home
>
> - Have you heard of gua sha? This is a traditional Chinese massage technique that involves gliding a smooth stone along the contours of the face. Over time, this simple at-home practice can help to lift jowls and create a more defined jaw. Here's how it's done:
>
> **1.** Apply a slippery serum that contains peptides or other skin-tightening ingredients.
>
> **2.** Take your gua sha stone and, starting underneath the eye, glide the tool in an outward and upward motion applying gentle pressure.
>
> **3.** Repeat this outward and upward stroke as you move down the face towards the jawline. You can increase the pressure when working with the lower face.
>
> **4.** Repeat this process for about five minutes on each side to create a temporary lifting effect, giving you a more refreshed and toned appearance.

# Hooded lids

If you're frequently told you look tired, hooded eyes might be to blame. Sagging skin around our peepers can make us appear older than we are – something none of us strive for! Read on to discover the tried-and-tested treatments that can deliver a bright, wide-eyed look, without going under the knife.

## What causes hooded lids?

We all get wrinkles with age, but not everyone will develop hooded lids. Here's why this sign of ageing hits some and not others:

**Family first**
You can blame your mum and dad. Genetics play a significant role in this common complaint. If a close family member has hooded lids, we're more likely to develop them too. Medical conditions that run through families (such as ptosis or blepharochalasis) can also increase our risk of hooded lids.

**Skin deep**
You know the drill – as the years tick by, the loss of supportive elastin and collagen leads to skin sagging and drooping. The muscles that support eyelids also weaken over time, contributing to a hooded look. Those with fair skin are more likely to develop sagging lids, as this skin type is more prone to sun damage and collagen breakdown.

## There's the rub

The skin around our eyes is delicate and prone to irritation. If we're always rubbing at our eyes (perhaps due to tiredness or allergies) this can contribute to droopiness.

## Treatments for hooded eyes

When skin has lost all elasticity, hooded lids can require surgical intervention. However, if we're quick to act, there's plenty that can be done to lift lids and avoid going under the knife.

### Sofwave™

This innovative treatment has FDA clearance for use in non-surgical brow lifts. When applied above and below the brow, as well as under the eye, it tightens and lifts the skin on lids as well as the whole eye area.

### Energy devices

Radiofrequency, ultrasound and laser therapy can be used to specifically target skin around the eyes. These treatments stimulate collagen production, leading to firmer skin.

### HIFES

High-intensity facial electromagnetic stimulation treatments can help to subtly lift forehead muscles, in turn improving the appearance of hooded eyes.

**Toxin Injections**

Carefully applied toxin injections can relax muscles that drag eyebrows down. This lifts the brows and opens up the eyes.

**Permanent makeup**

While permanent brow makeup (or microblading) can't technically lift hooded lids, it can give the illusion of an eye lift when drooping brows are cleverly repositioned.

---

### Try this at home

- Some eye creams can help to stimulate collagen production and tighten skin around the eyes. Look for ingredients such as retinol and peptides. While these creams are not likely to deliver dramatic results on their own, they can improve the texture and tone of skin and complement in-clinic interventions.

# Dark under-eye circles

Dark under-eye circles can get worse in later life but they don't discriminate. I've helped people of all ages and backgrounds achieve a brighter look.

## What causes dark under-eye circles?

Not all dark circles are created equal. Here are the most common causes to be aware of:

**Grey area**
Some dark circles are created by a build-up of excess skin pigmentation under the eye. This can happen if we rub our eyes often, spend too much time in the sun or have a skin condition such as eczema or allergic contact dermatitis. These pigment-related dark circles (also known as periorbital hyperpigmentation) are more common in people with darker skin tones.

**Clear as day**
Dark circles are more likely to appear as skin under our eyes becomes thinner and more translucent with age. This makes blood vessels more visible, giving skin a blue-ish or purple-ish tint. If we've lost fat from our under-eye area this can also create hollows and shadows that appear as dark circles.

**Home truths**

DNA can play an important role in the development of dark under-eye circles. If our close family members have dark circles, we are more likely to develop them too.

## Treatments for dark under-eye circles

From filler to radiofrequency, these non-surgical treatments make light work of brightening under-eyes.

### Filler

If under-eye hollows are creating darkness, hyaluronic acid filler injections can help to restore volume. In some, however, this hydrating ingredient can contribute to further fluid retention in the area, making dark circles worse. For this reason, I tend to recommend calcium hydroxyapatite (Radiesse) filler which restores volume without excess fluid.

### Microneedling with exosomes

This promising new treatment for dark under-eye circles combines the collagen-boosting effects of microneedling with a powerful exosome serum. Exosomes are natural molecules that are rich in growth factors and peptides that stimulate skin repair, reduce pigmentation, and improve skin thickness. Together, this dynamic duo can deliver a brighter under-eye in no time.

### Skin-boosting injections

Look out for polynucleotide injections– this powerful ingredient can tackle under-eye circles without causing any puffy fluid retention.

**Energy devices**
If skin transparency is the issue, radiofrequency, ultrasound, laser energy and Sofwave™ treatments can help to stimulate collagen for thicker, healthier skin.

**PRP**
Platelet-rich plasma therapy (also known as the 'vampire facial') can help to reduce the visibility of under-eye bags by stimulating collagen production and thickening skin. Natural growth factors are extracted from blood and then injected into problem areas for a boost in skin strength and brightness.

---

## Try this at home

- A healthy lifestyle can go a long way when it comes to brightening dark under-eyes. This means getting plenty of sleep, staying hydrated, limiting alcohol and ditching vapes and cigarettes. Your skin will thank you!

- Brightening eye creams can help to tackle pigmentation and enhance skin strength in this delicate area. Look for those that star vitamin C, peptides, retinol or brown algae.

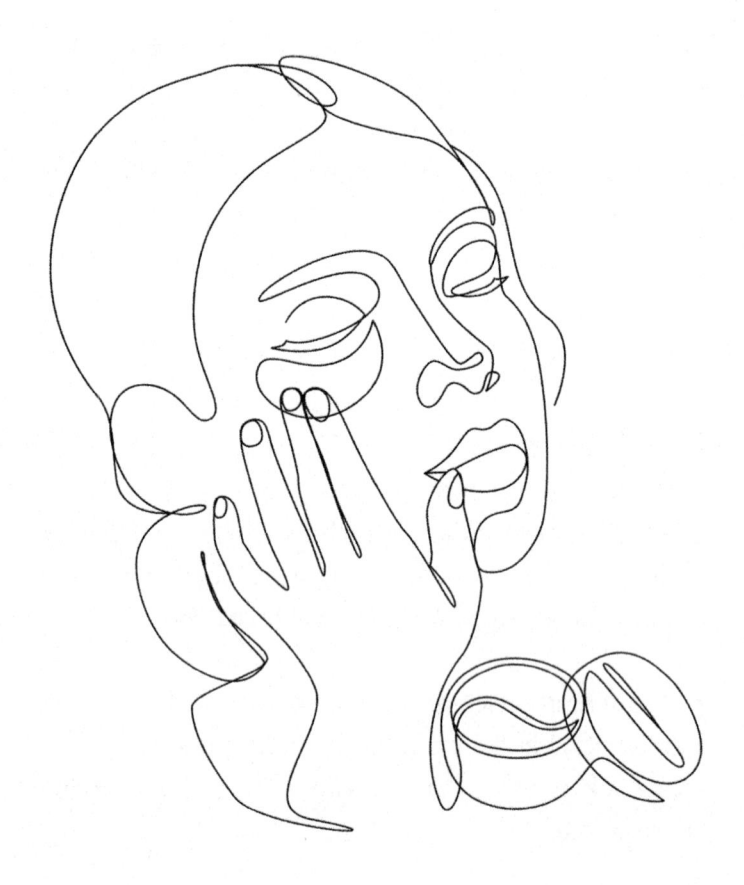

# Under-eye bags

Wouldn't it be lovely if shopping bags were the only bags in our lives? Sadly, under-eye bulges are a common ageing concern. While they can look like dark circles, bags appear for different reasons and require different treatments.

## What causes under-eye bags?

There are two types of under-eye bags: malar and festoons. Malar bags are patches of swelling that sit on the upper cheek, while festoons are folds of skin and under-eye muscle that appear as puffy bags. Here's what can make them more likely to appear:

**Blue genes**
It's that pesky DNA again. If our parents or grandparents have under-eye bags, we're more likely to develop them in later life.

**Peek-a-boo**
Sometimes facial fat can bulge out through a weak spot in the orbital septum – a thin membrane that normally keeps fat around the eyes in place.

**Age old**
Age-related changes in our skin (including a loss of skin strength and elastin) can contribute to under-eye bags.

## Treatments for under-eye bags

In cases where fat pads are particularly prominent, surgery may be the only way to completely erase under-eye bags. In less severe cases, however, non-surgical treatments can soften and smooth the area for a more youthful look. Here are my favourites:

**Energy devices**
Radiofrequency, ultrasound, laser and Sofwave™ treatments can help to stimulate collagen in skin under our eyes, reducing the appearance of bags.

**Skin-boosting injections**
Look for injections that contain polynucleotides. This super ingredient supports tissue regeneration and minimises under-eye bags. Steer clear of more hydrating ingredients (such as hyaluronic acid) as these can encourage fluid retention and exacerbate puffiness.

## Try this at home

- Taking steps to eat less salt can help to de-puff under-eye bags as excess sodium encourages fluid retention.

- Simple at-home facial massage techniques can help to drain excess fluid and soften bags. I do this each morning in the shower as the warm water allows fingers to glide more easily over skin:

**1.** Beginning at the bridge of your nose, use your middle and ring fingers to apply pressure in a rolling motion towards the outer corners of your eyes.

**2.** Be firm but careful not to pull or drag the skin. Do not lift your fingers as you move outward as maintaining continuous pressure is crucial to the drainage process.

**3.** Aim to direct your fingers towards the lymph glands located at the sides of your face. This helps drain away any excess fluid that has built up overnight, reducing puffiness and dark circles. Repeat this movement for a total of 3-5 times.

**4.** To achieve best results, head to my Instagram page (*@thebeautystudiomedispa*), where you'll find a video demonstration of this technique.

# Temporal veins

Have you ever noticed veins protruding around your temples? These are known as temporal veins and can become more prominent as we age.

## What causes temporal veins?

Age-related changes to our faces can make veins appear more prominent.

**Thick skin**
Our veins don't grow larger or thicker as we age – they simply become more visible due to our ageing skin. As we lose collagen, skin becomes thinner and more translucent. We may also lose facial fat, making veins more apparent.

**Not fair**
Temporal veins tend to be more visible against fair skin. Paler skin tones are also more vulnerable to sun damage and accelerated skin ageing, making prominent veins more likely to appear.

## Treatments for temporal veins

There's only one treatment I'd recommend for temporal veins, and it should always be performed by a medical professional.

**Vascular laser**
When light from this laser is absorbed by the blood vessel, the blood heats and coagulates. As a result, the vein is rendered inactive and is reabsorbed by the body. It should then disappear after approximately four weeks.

---

### Try this at home

- While we can't treat temporal veins at home, we can prevent them from growing more prominent with diligent daily application of a broad-spectrum SPF and collagen-boosting skincare ingredients such as peptides and retinol.

# Lip lines

Who doesn't love the beep of a barcode when buying yourself a special treat? Well, here's a barcode you're less likely to love – 'barcode' lines, also known as lip lines. These are the vertical wrinkles that gather around our pout with age.

## What causes lip lines?

For many, lip lines are one of the most concerning signs of ageing. Here's why they appear:

**Lip service**
In our younger years, lips are full and plump, thanks to plenty of pout-perfecting collagen. However, as levels of this protein decline, (from our late twenties onwards), lips can deflate, making wrinkles more likely to appear.

**Walk the line**
Women are more vulnerable to lip lines than men who have thicker skin, more oil glands, and coarse facial hair which offers protection. Women with fairer complexions are the most likely to develop lines and wrinkles around the mouth due to the lack of sun-protective melanin in skin.

**Up in smoke**
If we repeatedly use muscles around the mouth (while smoking or

using a straw, for example) we're likely to develop wrinkles as the years pass. Sun exposure can also damage skin around our lips, increasing our speed of ageing.

## Treatments for lip lines

*Banish barcode lines with these effective, non-surgical interventions.*

### Fractional $CO_2$ laser resurfacing
This laser treatment smooths wrinkles and reduces the appearance of lines. Clinical studies have shown that it can stimulate collagen production, which is essential for rejuvenating lips and making them look youthful and plump.

### Toxin injections
As with almost any wrinkles, toxin injections are a helpful tool here. When carefully administered around the mouth, the toxin relaxes surrounding muscles without impairing movement – don't worry, you'll still be able to smile, pout, talk and eat! But, by softening these micro muscles, we can prevent skin from wrinkling during mouth movements, making this both a preventative and remedial treatment.

### Hyaluronic acid filler
When injected along the lip line, filler can reduce wrinkles by supporting mouth muscles and preventing pursing. However, it's essential to avoid overfilling, as doing so can alter the lip's natural contour. Some fillers are designed specifically for the lip area, offering subtle enhancement while they also stimulate collagen production, restore elasticity, and provide hydration.

**Skin-boosting injections**
Look for hyaluronic acid injections that have been designed with lines above the mouth in mind. This inside-out skincare solution can help to soften creases.

**Energy devices**
Radiofrequency, Sofwave™, laser, and ultrasound therapies can help to stimulate collagen production in the lip area, softening lines.

**Microneedling with exosomes**
This two-for-one treatment does a brilliant job of stimulating collagen and elastin production for smoother, plumper skin. Exosomes are rich in growth factors which help skin regenerate itself from the inside-out – a truly natural approach for those not fond of filler.

**Permanent makeup**
This non-invasive treatment can add definition to the lip line, adding subtle volume (if desired) and a younger, smoother-looking lip.

## Try this at home

- Using a retinol-based serum each night can help stimulate natural collagen production.

- Apply a sunscreen of at least SPF 30 during the day to protect against sun damage. SPF lip balms can also help to protect delicate lip skin from UV rays.

# Crow's feet

Often one of the first signs of ageing, crow's feet are the fine lines and wrinkles that gather around the corners of eyes. They go by other names too, (such as 'laughter lines' or 'expression lines') thanks to the role our facial expressions play in their development.

## What causes crow's feet?

The delicate skin around our eyes is more vulnerable to signs of ageing than other areas of the face. Here's why crow's feet can appear:

### Face off

If we're of a generally happy demeanour, we're (unfortunately) more likely to develop crow's feet. Over time facial expressions such as smiling and laughing (but also squinting) can etch deep lines into delicate skin around eyes.

### Wrinkle in time

Yes – you guessed it – skin ageing makes any wrinkles more likely to appear and crow's feet are no different. Prolonged sun exposure without adequate protection can speed up the natural loss of collagen and elastin, leading to crow's feet before our time. Our DNA can also influence how quickly our skin ages and how defined our laughter lines are likely to be.

### Skin scaffolding

It's not just hamsters that have padded cheeks! Ours contain fat pads that provide support and volume to the midface. As we age, these can shrink or shift downwards, leaving skin around the eyes more prone to sagging and wrinkling.

## Treatments for crow's feet

So, what can be done to say bye-bye-birdie? Plenty. Here's my pick of the best evidence-based treatments.

### Toxin injections

Start here: toxin injections make light work of temporarily relaxing the muscles responsible for squinting and wrinkling around the eyes. This smooths out existing lines and prevents new ones from forming in the future. Results are enhanced when combined with other treatments that tighten and tone skin.

### Filler

Hyaluronic acid filler can help to plump and hydrate skin around eyes, minimising fine lines and wrinkles. Fillers can also be used to fill in any hollow areas around the eyes, further minimising the appearance of crow's feet.

### Energy devices

Radio frequency, ultrasound, Sofwave™ and laser therapies can help to improve skin texture by stimulating collagen production. This can have a positive effect on wrinkles. I recommend Sofwave ™ as its earned FDA-approval for the treatment of lines and wrinkles.

### Skin-boosting injections

These injections stimulate skin from the inside-out with ingredients such as polynucleotides or hyaluronic acid. They can assist in regenerating tissue and stimulating collagen to soften fine lines.

## Microneedling with exosomes

Microneedling treatments encourage collagen and elastin production by creating tiny microinjuries that trigger the skin's natural healing response. These microinjuries also allow healing exosomes to find their way into the deeper layers of skin where they support cellular repair. The result? Healthier, plumper, younger-looking skin.

## HIFES

Like a workout for the face, high-intensity facial electromagnetic stimulation technology can help to increase the size and firmness of muscles in our cheeks. This means cheeks better support skin around eyes, reducing sagging and preventing wrinkles.

---

### Try this at home

- Skin serums packed with retinoids, peptides, and antioxidants can help to improve collagen production and skin texture, minimising the appearance of crow's feet over time. Argireline is another ingredient to look out for: it's a peptide that's been shown to have a relaxing effect on dynamic wrinkle lines around eyes.

- Wear a minimum of SPF 30 daily and, on particularly sunny days, protect delicate skin around eyes with large sunglasses or a wide-brimmed hat.

- If your sight isn't what it used to be, don't skip a trip to the opticians. By getting our hands on the correct glasses (or contact lenses, if you don't fancy frames) we can avoid the constant squinting that leads to crow's feet.

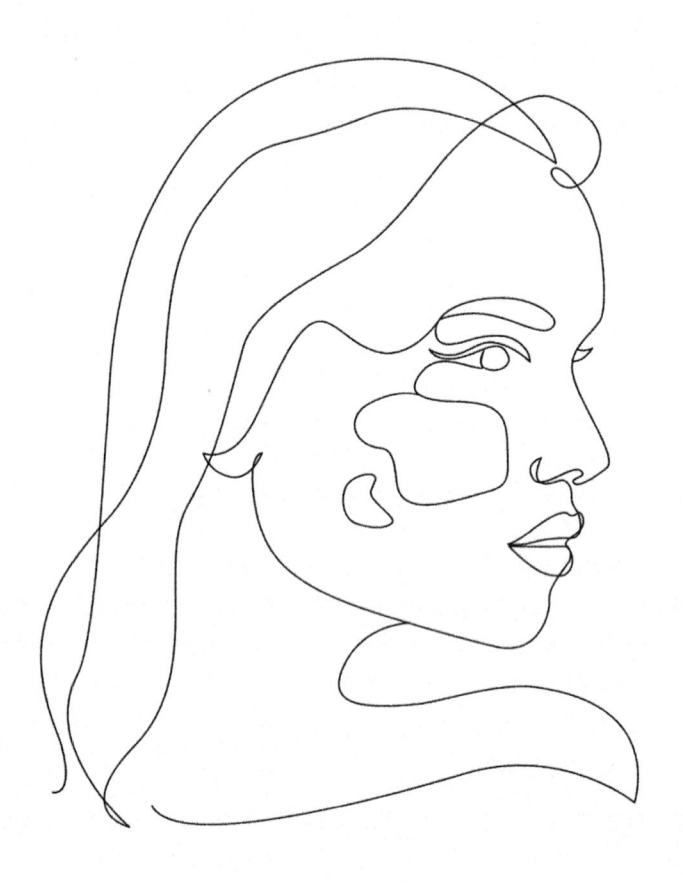

# Skin tone changes

We know we need to pile all skin-friendly colours of the rainbow on to our plates (from deep purple beetroots to bright red peppers) but we needn't welcome these colours onto our faces. As our blood vessels become more visible with age, skin can look increasingly red, purple or blue in places. Meanwhile, brown, orange and sallow yellow hues appear when our pigment-producing skin cells go awry.

We tend to associate signs of ageing with wrinkling and sagging but these skin tone changes account for 50% of the visible signs of getting on. This is good news as taking straightforward steps to develop a more even skin tone can make a dramatic difference to how we look from midlife onwards.

## What causes skin tone changes?

Skin tone changes occur thanks to a potent cocktail of genetic, lifestyle and environmental factors. Here's what you need to know:

**You're so vein**
If skin is looking blue, purple, red or even green in places, we can thank our increasingly visible blood vessels. These peek through because, as levels of collagen, elastin and youthful facial fat plummet, our skin structures become thinner and more translucent. We may also spot broken veins on the surface of skin – particularly around the cheeks and nose. Just as our bones grow more brittle with age, our veins also lose their suppleness. This stiffness hampers their function and they're more likely to permanently dilate.

### Here comes the sun

If, like me, your misspent youth featured sun beds and tanning oil, you're much more likely to see changes in your skin tone with age. UV rays accelerate the ageing process, contributing to the appearance of visible blood vessels as well as brown, orange and yellow hues.

### Game of life

Our daily choices and environment play an important role in the health of our skin. If we're more outdoorsy (frequently moving between the icy elements and sweltering central heating) this can challenge skin's resilience, promoting the appearance of broken veins. Smoking and drinking too much alcohol can also increase the accumulation of broken veins.

## Treatments for skin tone changes

There's lots we can do to treat visible facial veins and create a more even skin tone. Here's where to start:

### IPL

Intense pulsed light therapy is less powerful than laser and so is best for smaller veins. As with laser treatments, IPL heats and coagulates blood in offending veins, causing them to collapse and be absorbed by the body.

## Try this at home

- Skincare is the best defence against skin tone changes, helping to strengthen the skin barrier, improve elasticity and stave off less flattering hues. Here are the ingredients to look out for:

**Aescin** This anti-inflammatory and vasoconstrictive ingredient can help to minimise and shrink surface blood vessels.

**Botanical extracts** Natural anti-inflammatory extracts such as red vine leaf, arnica, and butcher's broom, work to improve microcirculation and reduce visible veins.

**Vitamin K** This vitamin can help reduce the appearance of broken capillaries and spider veins by strengthening vein walls and improving blood flow.

**Niacinamide (vitamin B3)** This increasingly popular ingredient works to improve the skin's barrier, reduce inflammation and enhance microcirculation, making it a good option for those hoping to reduce redness and vanish visible veins.

**Hyaluronic acid** You'll struggle to find a moisturiser, serum or mask that doesn't contain this hydrating hero. It's a great all-rounder that improves the health of skin, preventing skin tone changes from occurring.

**Sunscreen** Don't skip this step. Daily sunscreen use protects skin from UV damage, the biggest driver of visible veins and all aspects of skin ageing. When it comes to SPF, consistency is key so be sure to find a formula that sits well under make-up and that you enjoy wearing.

# Age spots & pigmentation

Age spots, also known as sun or liver spots, are the patches of dark or light brown pigment that appear on skin as we age. They can be found in different shapes and sizes and typically appear on areas of the body most often exposed to the sun, including the face, arms, and hands.

## What causes age spots and pigmentation?

From post-inflammatory pigmentation to sun spots and melasma, skin pigmentation can take lots of different forms. Understanding what's driving pigment in your skin is key to selecting the right treatment.

**Mr. Blue Sky**
Sun exposure is public enemy number one when it comes to pigmentation. UV rays damage skin cells which can lead to the overproduction of melanin, the pigment that gives skin its colour. Over time, this increased melanin can accumulate in certain areas, forming age spots. These rays can also encourage pigment to gather around a previous skin trauma such as a cut or acne spot – this is known as post-inflammatory pigmentation. UV damage can also worsen pigmentation that's triggered by hormone changes, such as melasma.

### In the blood

Sometimes pigmentation has its roots in nature not nurture. Our genes play a role in how susceptible we are to age spots with DNA mutations affecting how our skin responds to sunlight. If we have darker skin, for example, we're more likely to develop post-inflammatory pigmentation, while those with fair skin tones are more vulnerable to sun spots.

### Turn back time

As we age, our skin grows more vulnerable to pigmentation. While we are likely to have fewer pigment-producing skin cells (known as melanocytes) in our second half of life, those that remain get bigger. Unfortunately, these large melanocytes are more likely to distribute pigment unevenly, leading to age spots. Our skin also becomes less efficient at repairing damaged cells and so we are more susceptible to the long-term effects of sun damage.

## Treatments for sun spots and pigmentation

**For best results combine non-surgical treatments with at-home preventative care. Here's where to start:**

### IPL

Intense pulsed light therapy can minimise age spots by targeting melanin, the pigment responsible for skin colour. This high energy treatment also stimulates the skin's natural healing process, resulting in the production of new collagen and improved skin texture and tone.

### Skin peels

Skin peels, including chemical peels, can help to disappear pigmentation by removing the outer layers of damaged skin. This encourages the regeneration of new, less pigmented skin layers – leading to an overall reduction in pigmentation and an improvement in skin texture and tone.

**Skin-boosting injections**
Polynucleotide (PDRN) injections can help to reduce the inflammation that drives post-inflammatory hyperpigmentation and other pigmentation issues.

**Microneedling**
Microneedling creates helpful microinjuries that stimulate the skin's healing response and aid the absorption of any ingredients that are later applied. In cases of pigmentation, I'd recommend exosomes or a MesoFacial.

**MesoFacial**
In this popular treatment, microneedling is combined with a serum containing a blend of vitamins, minerals, and active ingredients designed to target melasma and hyperpigmentation. These include natural brighteners and tyrosinase inhibitors (a class of skin ingredients that block the enzyme responsible for pigment production). Expect happy, hydrated, plump and even-toned skin.

**Exosomes**
This cutting-edge ingredient contains growth factors and other bioactive molecules that influence the skin's immune response, reducing inflammation and helping to calm irritated skin. Exosomes are particularly helpful in cases of melasma or post-inflammatory hyperpigmentation where more aggressive treatments can make pigmentation worse.

**LED light therapy**
Commit to a course of non-invasive light therapy and you'll notice

reduced pigmentation and redness, as well as improved skin healing, tone and texture.

> ## Try this at home
>
> - A well-designed skincare routine can help to tackle sun spots and prevent pigmentation from appearing in the first place. These are the ingredients I'd recommend:
>
> **Retinoids** Retinoids are a one-stop-shop for treating pigmentation issues such as melasma, sun spots and post-inflammatory hyperpigmentation. They work by encouraging cell turnover and blocking pigment production.
>
> **Vitamin C** Research shows this antioxidant can limit UV damage, thereby slowing signs of ageing and preventing pigmentation. It can also lighten and brighten existing pigmentation.
>
> **Arbutin** Arbutin is a tyrosinase inhibitor that is often found in skin-lightening cosmetics.
>
> **Kojic acid** This fungi extract, blocks pigment production – a truly magic mushroom!
>
> **Azelaic acid** While more commonly used as an acne treatment, this skin-soothing acid can also help to block pigment production.
>
> **Liquorice extract** Liquorice can help to lighten and brighten dark spots by blocking the production of skin pigment.

## A NOTE ON HYDROQUINONE

Hydroquinone is a well-known pigmentation-buster that was once the go-to ingredient for treating hyperpigmentation. However, due to concerns over safety and side effects, the ingredients listed on the previous page are more commonly used and should be our first port of call.

# Facial flushing & redness

Pretty pink cheeks are a sign of youth, but when redness spreads down the cheeks, onto the neck or across the nose, facial flushing can take a toll on self-esteem and confidence. But we don't need to slather ourselves in increasingly high coverage foundation – instead, let's tackle the root causes of redness to restore skin confidence.

## What causes facial flushing and redness?

When we flush, blood vessels dilate below the skin's surface as blood rushes to our increasingly rosy complexion. Here's why this can happen:

**The change**
Hormonal changes during perimenopause can wreak havoc on the body's temperature regulation system, resulting in infamous menopausal hot flushes – a prickly heat that spreads across the body and up onto the face. For this reason, we're much more likely to experience repeated facial flushing in midlife.

**Hot stuff**
Eating spicy foods, drinking alcohol and taking certain medications can all lead to facial flushing.

**Rosacea**

Rosacea is a chronic inflammatory condition which can begin with flushing and escalate to bumps, pimples, and chronic redness.

## Treatments for facial flushing and redness

Ready to put a stop to redness once and for all? Here are the treatments to look out for at your local clinic:

**Near infrared lasers**
The standout treatment for redness, near infrared lasers target the dilated blood vessels that cause flushing. The near infrared light heats and coagulates blood without harming surrounding skin. This soothes redness and minimises the appearance of rosacea and spider veins.

**LED light therapy**
This non-invasive treatment reduces inflammation, calms redness, promotes circulation, stimulates collagen production, and enhances the skin barrier. The result? A more even skin tone and less noticeable redness.

**Microneedling with exosomes**
Exosomes are a cutting-edge ingredient that contain growth factors and other bioactive molecules that influence the skin's immune response. They can soothe inflammation, calm irritation and bring down areas of redness.

**IPL**
Intense pulsed light therapy can minimise redness by targeting haemoglobin, the pigment that gives blood its red colour. This high energy treatment also stimulates the skin's natural healing process – think improved skin texture and tone, as well as increased collagen production.

## Try this at home

- Look out for skincare ingredients such as piperonyl glucose, sea whip, and honokitiol, which offer targeted relief for redness.

- If menopausal hot flushes are to blame for redness, hormone replacement therapy can vanish this bothersome symptom (see more information on p.27). If HRT is not for you, seek the support of your GP – there are other treatments available.

# Common age-related skin blemishes

As we move through life our skin shows all sorts of signs of wear and tear – from seborrheic keratosis to skin tags and actinic keratosis. Here's how to treat these common skin concerns:

## Seborrheic keratosis

Typically brown, black, or light tan in appearance, seborrheic keratosis is a common, non-cancerous skin growth that tends to appear in middle age and older adults. They often have a waxy, scaly, slightly elevated appearance and are most frequently found on the face, neck, chest, and back. In most cases, they're genetic, though spending too much time in the sun can also magic them into existence.

**THE SOLUTION:** You can freeze these benign growths off with liquid nitrogen (known as cryotherapy) or zap them with a small probe (cauterisation).

## Skin tags

Like miniature flaps, skin tags are soft, benign growths. They're a byproduct of skin friction, and so are most often found where the skin folds – including the armpits, groin, neck, and under the breasts. Skin tags are usually the same colour as the surrounding skin or slightly darker. They tend to run in families and appear during times of hormonal upheaval such as pregnancy and menopause.

**THE SOLUTION:** As with seborrheic keratosis, skin tags can be quickly frozen or zapped off with a cryotherapy or cauterisation treatment.

## Actinic keratosis

Characterised by rough, scaly patches on the skin, actinic keratosis typically appears on sun-exposed areas such as the scalp, face, ears, neck, backs of hands, forearms, and chest. These patches are more common in those with sun-sensitive fair skin and are considered precancerous – so, if left untreated, may potentially develop into squamous cell carcinoma, a form of skin cancer.

**THE SOLUTION:** Due to the pre-cancerous nature of actinic keratosis, treatments should always be conducted by a medical professional. Interventions may include cryotherapy, prescription creams, laser or photodynamic therapy – a medical treatment which combines a light-sensitive drug with a specific type of light that can destroy abnormal cells.

## Lines and wrinkles

We've covered specific wrinkles in previous chapters (from marionette lines to crow's feet) but many experience more generalised skin-wrinkling that can affect all areas of the face. As collagen breaks down, we might start to notice this as a cross-hatched texture on skin. This is more common in individuals with fair skin and those who've spent lots of time in the sun.

**THE SOLUTION:** Sofwave™ is the leading evidence-based treatment for lines and wrinkles (it's earned FDA-approval for this purpose). Microneedling, ablative lasers and skin-boosting injections can also deliver smoothing results.

# Visible pores

It's not just those with oily skin that experience larger, more visible pores: as we get older, our skin undergoes several changes that can make pores more pronounced.

## What causes visible pores?

Ageing skin can emphasise and enlarge pores – here's what you need to know:

**Spring in your step**
We lose collagen and elastin with age, leaving skin less bouncy and more prone to sagging – a process that can happen much more quickly if we spend too much time in the sun. When skin sags, pores appear larger.

**Oil change**
We're encouraged to wash our faces daily for good reason! The oil naturally produced by the skin can mix with dead cells and become trapped in pores. This clogging effect stretches the pores and makes them more noticeable. This becomes more of a problem during menopause when hormonal fluctuations can drive excess oil production.

## How to treat visible pores

We don't have pore-shrinking technology (yet!) but collagen-stimulating treatments can help to tighten and tone skin, making pores less visible. Here are the best picks:

**Microneedling with exosomes**
Microneedling treatments encourage collagen and elastin production by creating tiny microinjuries that trigger the skin's natural healing response. These microinjuries allow exosomes into the deeper layers of skin where they support cellular repair and improve skin texture and elasticity for tiny looking pores.

**Chemical peels**
Salicylic or lactic acid peels are powerful exfoliators – removing dead skin cells and promoting new cell growth. This can help minimise the appearance of large pores.

**HydraFacial**
While this affordable treatment doesn't technically reduce pore size, it can clean out the pores and makes them appear smaller.

**Fractional laser**
This powerful laser treatment can help to resurface skin, stimulate collagen production and minimise the appearance of large pores.

**Fractional radiofrequency**
A multi-tasking hero, fractional radiofrequency combines the benefits of microneedling with radiofrequency energy. The result? Smoother, tighter-looking skin with minimised pores.

### Try this at home

- Encourage speedy cell renewal with exfoliating skincare ingredients such as retinol, lactic acid and salicylic acid.

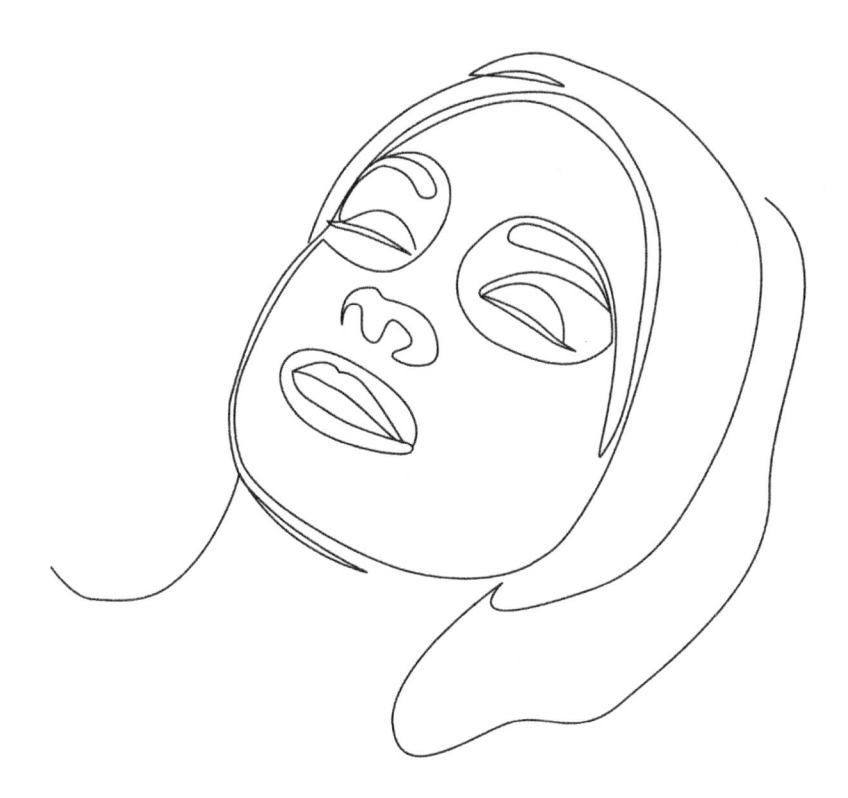

# Ageing hands

Even though they're just as on show as our face, we often don't give our hands the TLC they deserve until lines and loose skin become visible. It's about time we changed this...

## What causes ageing hands?

Our hands are more vulnerable to the signs of ageing than other areas of the body – here's why:

**Out and about**
Our hands are rarely covered and so fall victim to sun exposure and the wrinkles, loss of firmness, and age spots that follow. Skin on the backs of our hands is also thinner, leaving it more susceptible to damage, dehydration, loss of elasticity, and the development of fine lines and wrinkles.

**Wear and tear**
How often are your hands completely still? Daily living requires that our mitts are in constant motion and this repeated use can lead to creases, lines, and wrinkles. Our hands are also more likely to encounter harsh chemicals, such as detergents, cleaning agents, and soaps, than other areas of the body. These chemicals strip the natural oils from the skin, leading to dryness, irritation, and accelerated ageing.

# Treatments for ageing hands

Need a helping hand? Try these non-surgical treatments:

**Fillers**
Hyaluronic acid filler can restore volume to our hands, plumping up thinning skin and reducing the appearance of wrinkles and fine lines. Fillers can also help to camouflage visible veins and tendons, creating a smoother, more youthful look.

**Skin-boosting injections**
Stimulate collagen production and regenerate tissue from the inside-out with polynucleotide or hyaluronic acid injections.

**Skin peels**
Not just for the face! A chemical peel does what it says on the tin – it peels away the skin's outer layer. This helps to improve the texture and tone of our hands and fade any tell-tale age spots.

**Laser therapy**
Laser treatments, such as fractional laser resurfacing, can boost collagen production and help fade discolouration, resulting in smoother, more even-toned skin.

**IPL**
Intense pulsed light therapy can be used to target signs of ageing on hands, such as wrinkles, uneven skin texture, and age spots.

**Microneedling**
By stimulating the body's natural healing processes and giving collagen levels a boost, microneedling can reduce the appearance of fine lines and wrinkles and leave our hands looking better than ever.

**Sclerotherapy**

If visible veins are the cause of your hand woes, try sclerotherapy. During this procedure, a sclerosing solution is injected into the veins, causing them to collapse and disappear over time for a more youthful look. This treatment should always be carried out by a medical professional.

---

### Try this at home

- Show your hands as much love as your face during skincare rituals. Skin heroes such as retinol, antioxidants, and alpha hydroxy acids (AHAs) can help to stimulate collagen production, improve the tone and texture of our hands, and fade age spots. And don't skip SPF! Our hardworking mitts need protection too.

- Apply a moisturising hand cream after every handwash for an extra burst of hydration.

# PART THREE

## Your Non-surgical Journey

You should now know how to take care of your skin at home, as well as the very best, evidence-based treatments for any specific ageing concerns you might have. In this third section, we'll be filling in the missing piece of the non-surgical puzzle – a brilliant aesthetic therapist.

In the following pages, I'll share everything to keep in mind while choosing a reputable practitioner and progressing your aesthetic goals. Let's dive in.

# How to choose a good clinic

Take a stroll down any high street and you'll likely find a beauty and aesthetics salon brimming with high-tech services. Picking a reputable salon and therapist is key – you're quite literally putting your face in their hands. These need to be hands you can trust.

By asking the right questions and doing your research ahead of time you can keep your skin safe. Here's where to start:

**Check out reviews:** Just as you would for a restaurant or hotel, look at their Google or Facebook reviews. These should give honest accounts of previous clients' experiences.

**Look at prices:** Generally, if a treatment price seems too good to be true, it probably is! Compare your local salon's prices to the guidelines I've included in the treatment index (from p127) – anything well below this figure should ring alarm bells.

**Look for authenticity:** As a MediSpa owner, I receive almost daily emails from 'vendors' offering cheaply imported equipment. These are replicas of well-known devices, sometimes offered at one twentieth of the price of the real thing.

These cheaper alternatives come with a significant drop in quality, and (perhaps even more worrying) the therapists are given no training from the seller about how to use the device.

No reputable high street salon or MediSpa would opt for these dubious devices. As a client, I advise you look up the exact name of the treatment you're considering. If it's not listed on the website, do ask the clinic for the details.

I've included reputable brands to look out for in the treatment index (if a salon is using these, it's a very good sign). But buyer beware: sometimes imitation devices have minor variations in the name – for instance, clinics offering the genuine treatment may use all capital letters, while the fake version might be in lowercase or have a single letter changed. A good example of this is HydroFacial, a cheap copy of the popular HydraFacial. These subtle differences are red flags, so it's important to pay attention to the details to ensure you'll receive the authentic treatment.

**Review the clinic's therapists:** I cannot overstate the importance of choosing a clinic that has highly trained and experienced staff. Just as important as the devices used, the expertise of the staff will impact the quality of the treatment you receive. An experienced therapist will also be able to better diagnose and treat a wide range of skin concerns and recommend the most accurate and effective treatments.

While you can't go browsing CVs, a clinic's website can often indicate their commitment (or lack of commitment) to staff training and development. By prioritising staff education, a clinic demonstrates its dedication to maintaining high standards.

---

### Variety is key

Usually, no single procedure will meet all your aesthetic goals. For instance, while fillers may offer more defined cheekbones, they will not improve the look and overall quality of skin.

Selecting a therapist with plenty of tools in their toolbox, and who can offer a wide range of services and solutions, will help you achieve optimal outcomes.

# Watch out for perception drift

Before you head off to your local clinic, I want you to keep 'perception drift' in mind. When embarking on a pro-ageing journey with high-tech treatments such as toxin injections and fillers, it's important to keep a balanced perspective.

Perception drift refers to the gradual – and often subconscious – shift in our perception of how we look. If not properly managed, this loss of perspective can lead some to make more and more dramatic alterations to their appearance. This quest for 'perfection' can leave us looking less and less like ourselves as we lose the unique features that define our natural beauty and make us who we are.

## The initial excitement

Picture this: you start with a single treatment – a couple of toxin injections to smooth out forehead wrinkles or a little filler to plump up thinning lips. The results are striking, providing an immediate boost to your confidence and a sense of renewed youthfulness. This initial 'wow factor' and flurry of compliments from friends creates a buzz that encourages thoughts of further treatments.

As time progresses, the initial thrill of the treatment starts to wane. The subtle changes that once brought so much joy no longer seem as impactful – and this is where perception drift can begin to take hold. Your idea of what looks normal and youthful starts to shift, and what was once considered an ideal appearance might now feel inadequate.

So, to regain that buzz, you opt for additional fillers or more frequent toxin injections. The satisfaction returns, but it's short-lived – maintaining that same level of perceived youthfulness requires increasingly invasive measures as we age. The treatments that once felt like minor adjustments can escalate into more significant alterations, such as extensive plastic surgery.

Mental health implications aside, the sad truth is that the pursuit of eternal youth can paradoxically lead to a less youthful appearance. Too much filler can create unnatural puffiness, while excessive toxin injections can lead to a frozen, expressionless face. Surgical interventions, if not approached with caution, can result in drastic changes that take us further away from our aesthetic goals.

## Maintaining balance and perspective

**To avoid falling into the trap of perception drift, keep these guidelines in mind:**

**Set realistic goals:** Clearly define what you hope to achieve with your treatments. Aim for subtle enhancements that maintain your natural look.

**Seek professional guidance:** Choose experienced practitioners who prioritise natural results and can help you understand the limitations and risks of each procedure.

**Monitor your progress:** Regularly review your appearance with a critical eye, possibly with the help of trusted friends or family members who can provide honest feedback.

**Take breaks:** Allow time between treatments to assess whether further procedures are genuinely necessary or if they are being driven by a desire for that temporary high.

**Prioritise overall wellbeing:** Remember that true beauty is holistic. Focus on a healthy lifestyle, including proper nutrition, exercise, and skincare, to complement your cosmetic treatments.

By acknowledging perception drift, we can make informed decisions that align with our long-term aesthetic goals and overall wellbeing. The key is to enhance our natural beauty without losing sight of who we are, maintaining a youthful appearance that feels both authentic and sustainable.

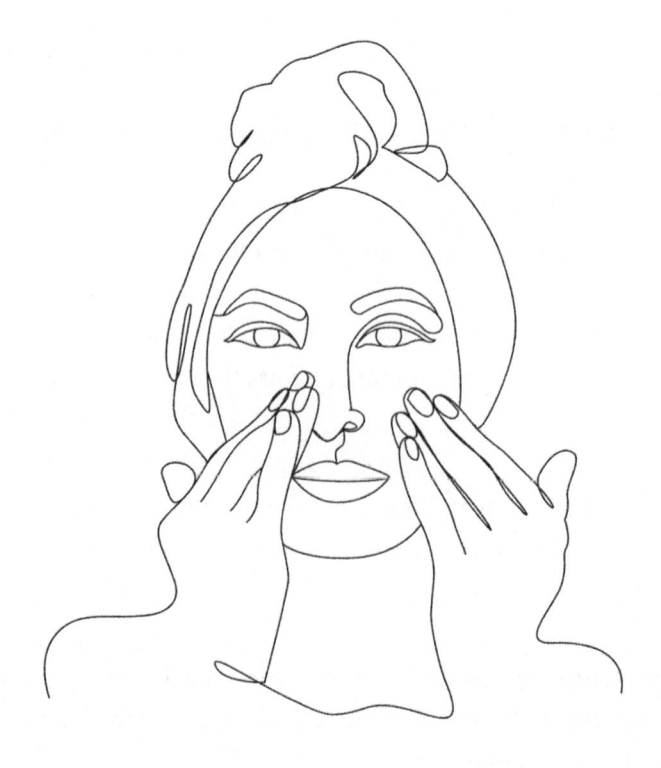

# Navigating aesthetic treatments after cancer

At my MediSpa, we often welcome clients who have medical conditions or have undergone cancer treatment and are now cancer-free.

For many who have endured the challenges of a serious illness, starting a new skin treatment or non-surgical intervention is a significant step towards feeling better and reclaiming a sense of normality.

Unfortunately, MediSpa clinics often have to turn these women away or offer a very limited treatment menu due to insurance policies which require clients to be in remission or cancer-free for five years. In some cases, treatments are only permitted if a letter from your consultant confirms that it's safe to proceed.

Client safety must always come first, but these restrictions are often upsetting for both the client and the MediSpa staff. This was the case for a friend of mine who treated herself to a spa weekend after finally hearing those long-awaited words – "you're cancer-free!" Upon arrival at the spa she undressed, got ready for her massage and disclosed her medical history only to be told that they couldn't proceed because of her history of cancer. The experience was so distressing that she packed her bags and left.

If you are still under the care of your consultant, I suggest asking them for a letter of clearance for any future treatments you may wish to pursue. Once you are no longer under their care, obtaining such a letter can become more difficult, and GPs are often reluctant to provide the necessary documentation. Even treatments as seemingly simple as a massage can require a note from your doctor. It might be helpful to request a letter that allows for massages and facials, as well as non-surgical ultrasound, laser and radiofrequency therapies to cover all bases.

During your cancer treatment, these considerations may not seem like a priority – but they can play a helpful role in your later recovery. Most consultants recognise the importance of feeling good about yourself and are usually willing to support you on your journey.

# Looking ahead to your skincare journey

As we draw near the end of this book, let's take a moment to reflect. We've explored the world of non-surgical skincare, investigated the science behind skin ageing, delved into the importance of wellbeing and a positive mindset, and uncovered powerful tools that can help you age gracefully. I hope you feel empowered by the knowledge you've gained.

The world of skincare is ever evolving, and new innovations are emerging all the time. Now that you understand the foundations of non-surgical skin rejuvenation, I encourage you to try new things – whether it's a cutting-edge treatment or a new product. Don't forget to explore the treatment index (p.126) for further information on the treatments and technologies I outlined in Part Two.

Ageing is a natural process, and, with the right approach, you can look and feel your best at every stage of life. The small, deliberate actions you take each day (whether it's applying SPF, scheduling monthly facials, or maintaining a healthy lifestyle) are what make the difference over time. It's not about drastic changes or overnight transformations – well, maybe sometimes – but the non-surgical techniques and treatments we've discussed are most effective when they become a consistent part of your routine. Remember – your skin reflects the time and care you invest in it.

Take your next steps with confidence. Perhaps you'll schedule your first skin consultation at your local MediSpa, incorporate new skincare practices into your daily routine, or simply make a commitment to prioritise self-care. The choice is yours. As Michelle Obama said: "We need to do a better job of putting ourselves higher on our own 'to do' list."

Your journey to ageing well is ongoing, and every small step contributes to your overall wellbeing.

For tips on ageing well and to stay up to date with the latest trends, follow my MediSpa clinic on Instagram: @thebeautystudiomedispa.

I look forward to meeting you!

Sandy

# PART FOUR

## Treatment Index

In this fourth and final section, I will be answering any questions you might have before booking a non-surgical treatment. How much will it cost? Will it hurt? When will I see results? Don't worry, I've got you covered.

This is by no means an exhaustive list of every available technology, but I have included the most popular and well-researched treatments you are likely to encounter.

And, as I explained in Part Three, it's important to understand the specific brand of technology your local clinic is offering. That's why, in the following pages, I've also detailed the reputable brands to look out for – this will keep you safe and ensure you are likely to get great results. Let's dive in.

# Skin peels

**BEST FOR:** Brightening dull skin; reducing pigmentation, age spots and melasma; enhancing skin texture; minimising pore size; reducing fine lines and wrinkles.

## How do skin peels work?

Peels use acids to dissolve the natural bonds that keep dead skin cells attached to the skin's surface. This exfoliation reveals the fresh skin underneath, leading to a brighter appearance and more even skin tone. With dead skin cells sloughed off, our skin is better able to absorb our skincare products, too – and so anti-ageing ingredients (such as retinol and peptides) work harder for us.

## Are there different types?

Different acids are used in skin peels depending on the skin concern and degree of peeling required. Light and superficial peels aim to refresh the skin, while medium and deep peels are typically designed to address more profound skin issues, such as wrinkles and scarring.

## Which peel is right for me?

The two most effective acids used in progressive peels are lactic and salicylic acid.

**Lactic acid**

This multi-tasking hero hydrates while it gently exfoliates. Its larger molecular size allows for slower skin penetration, making it an ideal choice for those with sensitive skin or who are new to chemical peels. It will leave your skin hydrated, while also improving elasticity and reducing wrinkle depth.

**Salicylic acid**

This acid is brilliant for pigmentation-prone skin. By gently removing the skin's upper layer (and reducing melanin accumulation), it lightens hyperpigmentation, age spots, and melasma for a more even skin tone. Research also suggests that salicylic acid can help to protect skin against UV damage and promote DNA repair. A powerful pro-ageing ally!

---

### The progressive peeling approach

Deep chemical peels use the most powerful acids for the most dramatic results, but they also come with a set of risks. Top of the list, is the risk of post-inflammatory hyperpigmentation (PIH) which can lead to long-term skin discolouration.

Deep peels also come with more downtime (think red, peeling skin) and an increased risk of long-term skin injury, including infections and scarring. That's why I always recommend a 'progressive peeling' strategy.

This approach involves using milder acids over multiple sessions, each time gradually increasing the strength and treatment duration. The end result is just as impressive but we dramatically reduce the risk of complications – it's a no-brainer!

# THE FACTS

**What to expect**
Don't worry, skin peels aren't as scary as they sound! The therapist will apply the acid mixture to your skin and leave it to sit for a short time. After this, the acid is neutralised and the therapist will usually apply a soothing face mask, followed by sunscreen. Some peels can be applied and left on overnight, with the acid gradually neutralising itself.

**Does it hurt?**
During a mild progressive peel, you might notice some light skin-stinging or tingling. Deeper acid peels can be more uncomfortable, but shouldn't be painful.

**Is there any downtime?**
You may notice pink, tight-feeling skin and light skin peeling for between one to five days, depending on the strength of the peel. A progressive peel approach will keep downtime to an absolute minimum.

**When will I see results?**
After seven to ten days, skin will appear smooth, radiant and hydrated as the fresh new skin cells are revealed. Multiple peels are needed to tackle skin concerns such as pigmentation.

**How long do results last?**
Results last between six to twelve months depending on the strength of a skin peel and how many treatments you commit to.

**Recommended brands:** AlumierMD, Skinceuticals, ZO Skin Health

**Price:** From £90

# Radiofrequency

**BEST FOR:** Tightening skin; reducing fine lines and wrinkles.

## How do radiofrequency treatments work?

No FM tuning involved here: radiofrequency (RF) is a non-invasive technology used to tighten skin and reduce wrinkles. The RF energy generates heat which is used to slowly raise the temperature of the dermis (the skin's deepest layer) to approximately 41°C. This heat triggers the body's natural healing response and the production of plumping collagen, elastin, and other helpful skin-boosters. The result? Tighter, smoother, more elastic skin.

## THE FACTS

**What to expect**
The therapist will thoroughly cleanse your skin, before applying a conductive gel. A wand that emits RF waves is then massaged over the area for approximately 30-45 minutes.

**Does it hurt?**
Your skin is likely to feel very hot, but the therapist will keep the wand moving so that it remains comfortable.

**Is there any downtime?**
The downtime required after an RF treatment is minimal. You may experience redness and slight swelling for up to 24 hours, but these symptoms resolve quickly in most cases.

**When will I see results?**
Don't expect immediate results. The benefits of RF appear gradually over a period of weeks and months as skin repairs and remodels itself. For best results a course of four to six treatments is recommended.

**How long do results last?**
Results last for up to a year, depending on the condition of skin and how many treatments you commit to. Periodical maintenance treatments can help to preserve results.

**Recommended brands:** Exion, Pollogen Legend, Forma, EndyMed, Lynton Dynamix

**Price:** From £100 per session

# Fractional radiofrequency

**BEST FOR:** Tightening skin; minimising visible pores; enhancing skin texture; softening lines and wrinkles.

## How does FRF work?

Fractional radiofrequency (FRF) – also known as radiofrequency microneedling – combines the benefits of microneedling with RF energy for maximum skin rejuvenation.

The specialised handpiece is covered in needles that make microinjuries in the skin and emit RF energy as they go. This heat energy gets deep into the dermis (without damaging skin's visible outer layers) to activate the body's healing processes. The result? Lots of lovely collagen and elastin production for tighter, smoother, more youthful-looking skin.

> ## Is FRF right for me?
>
> FRF is generally suitable for all skin tones, but those with darker skin tones need to be more cautious. A good therapist can recommend a device with insulated needle tips to reduce the risk of post-inflammatory hyperpigmentation. Similarly, lower energy settings can also be used to further minimise this risk. The devil is in the details.

## THE FACTS

**What to expect**
The therapist will thoroughly cleanse your skin, before applying a numbing cream to minimise discomfort. Then they'll get to work with the microneedling handpiece. This looks a bit like a tattoo pen with around 36 fine needles that penetrate skin at depths ranging from 0.5 mm to 3mm. The treatment usually takes between 30-60 minutes.

**Does it hurt?**
The level of discomfort can vary depending on the specific technology used. Some newer FRF treatments, like Exion, make use of artificial intelligence in the needle tip (yes, really!) to adjust RF power, pulse duration and needling speed. This innovation helps reduce pain without sacrificing the results.

**Is there any downtime?**
You may notice pink skin or subtle pinprick marks for up to a week after the treatment – nothing that need keep you locked away indoors!

**When will I see results?**
You can expect immediate improvements in skin brightness, as well as the appearance of pores and scars. Over a period of weeks and months, you'll also benefit from increased collagen and elastin production which shows up as tighter, smoother skin. For best results, a course of four treatments spaced about a month apart is usually recommended. The full effects will be seen approximately three months after your last session.

**How long do results last?**
Results last up to a year, depending on the condition of your skin and how many treatments you commit to. Periodical maintenance treatments can help to preserve results.

**Recommended brands:** Exion, Secret RF, Focus Dual

**Price:** From £500

# High-intensity focused ultrasound (HIFU)

**BEST FOR:** Tightening skin; contouring the face; reducing fine lines and wrinkles.

## How does HIFU work?

High-intensity focused ultrasound (HIFU) technology shares the same goal as radiofrequency treatments: they both stimulate the body's natural healing and regenerative processes but do this in slightly different ways.

While radiofrequency waves transmit heat energy, HIFU emits soundwaves at frequencies higher than humans can hear. These high-pitched sounds travel deep into skin where they're absorbed and converted into heat.

This heat inflicts controlled damage to the skin, triggering the body's healing response. Over time, the production of skin-plumping proteins (collagen and elastin) ramps up and we see tighter, smoother skin.

## Get focused

A word to the wise: there are lots of worryingly cheap HIFU devices on the market, which can't accurately monitor our skin's temperature during the treatment. This is not ideal as, if temperatures get too hot, we risk melting our facial fat.

You can avoid this by opting for micro-focused ultrasound technology, which comes with high-resolution imaging so your therapist can accurately tweak the intensity and depth of the ultrasound energy. This keeps you and your skin safe.

## THE FACTS

**What to expect**
The therapist will thoroughly cleanse your skin before applying a gel. The HIFU device is then placed against the skin to work its magic.

**Does it hurt?**
They say there's no gain without pain and, unfortunately, ultrasound treatments can be uncomfortable. Expect a sharp, zapping sensation, alongside intense heat –manageable but not relaxing. Micro-focused ultrasound treatments are less uncomfortable and taking a painkiller before a session can help. Topic anaesthetic can also be applied to make the treatment more comfortable.

**Is there any downtime?**
There's typically no downtime required after a HIFU treatment. Mild redness, swelling, and tenderness may occur in the treated area, but these effects usually subside within 24 hours.

**When will I see results?**
You may notice some immediate tightening, but the full results are clear after three months as new collagen is produced. Clinical studies show that collagen, elastin and hyaluronic acid continue to increase for up to nine months, making this treatment a gift that keeps on giving. For best results, one to two sessions spaced one to three months apart is usually recommended

**How long do results last?**
Results typically last twelve months depending on the condition of your skin and how many treatments you commit to.

**Recommended brands:** Ultherapy, Ultraformer 111

**Price:** From £2,000

# Parallel beam ultrasound (Sofwave™)

**BEST FOR:** Lifting hooded lids and drooping brows; softening fine lines and wrinkles; sculpting the jawline; improving the appearance of 'turkey neck'; tightening and lifting jowls.

Every now and then, a new technology emerges that captures my attention and gets those 'spidery senses' tingling. Sofwave™ is an ultrasound-based treatment, but it takes an innovative approach that's set to revolutionise the non-surgical skin space.

## How does Sofwave™ work?

Whereas HIFU delivers tiny dots of ultrasound energy into the skin, Sofwave™ employs a unique parallel beam approach. Put simply, seven parallel beams of ultrasound energy penetrate the skin reaching an optimal depth of 1.5 mm. What does this mean for your face? You'll notice significant improvements after just one session.

Sofwave™ stands out from the pack as the only non-invasive treatment that's received FDA approval for tightening skin under the chin and treating hooded eyelids, a drooping brow, sagging neck skin, fine lines and wrinkles.

## THE FACTS

**What to expect**
Prior to treatment, your therapist will apply a topical anaesthetic to skin and leave that to work its magic for thirty minutes. The Sofwave™ applicator head is then placed against the skin and moved across the face – first in one direction, and then the opposite direction.

**Does it hurt?**
You'll notice a heating sensation that builds in intensity but it's tolerable.

**Is there any downtime?**
You won't experience any redness or downtime.

**When will I see results?**
You'll likely notice minor improvements to the tightness and tone of skin immediately. However, the full effects are evident after nine to twelve weeks.

**How long do results last?**
Results last between twelve to eighteen months.

**Recommended brands:** Sofwave™ is currently the only brand offering this trade-marked technology.

**Price:** From £2,000 for a full face and neck treatment

# High-intensity facial electromagnetic stimulation (HIFES)

**BEST FOR:** Lifting jowls; sculpting the cheeks and jawline; facial contouring; creating a natural facelift effect.

One of the main reasons people choose to go under the knife is to have a face lift. But, you can achieve a lifting effect without surgery and high-intensity facial electromagnetic stimulation (HIFES) is one of the best treatments for this purpose.

## How does HIFES work?

The high intensity electromagnetic energy stimulates rapid muscle contractions in our facial muscles – like a workout for the face! These repeated contractions grow and tone our facial muscles, leading to a more lifted and youthful-looking face.

## THE FACTS

**What to expect**
Each HIFES treatment lasts twenty minutes. Your therapist will place applicators onto specific areas of the face to target muscle groups in the forehead, cheeks, and under the chin.

**Does it hurt?**
It's a strange sensation, but not at all painful.

**Is there any downtime?**
As the treatment is non-invasive, there's no downtime required – a definite boost to its appeal!

**When will I see results?**
You'll notice immediate results, but the full benefit can be seen after six to twelve weeks.

**How long do results last?**
Results last for up to a year with a maintenance treatment required every six months.

**Recommended brands:** EMFACE (this device combines HIFES with radiofrequency for a 2-in-1 treatment)

**Price:** From £400

# Laser

**BEST FOR:** Reducing fine lines and wrinkles; improving skin tone and texture; addressing pigmentation; minimising the appearance of veins; tightening skin.

There are two main types of laser used in cosmetic treatments: non-ablative and ablative. While both stimulate collagen production, non-ablative lasers achieve this by heating the underlying skin layers, whereas ablative lasers remove the outer layer of the skin.

## Non-ablative lasers

Non-ablative lasers are a safe, comfortable, and less invasive alternative to ablative lasers. They are ideal for skin that isn't showing advanced signs of ageing (think deep lines, severe sagging or dark pigmentation) and can help to soften fine lines and wrinkles as well as improve mild to moderate skin sagging, hyperpigmentation, redness, and acne scars. Non-ablative lasers can also slow down the ageing process and prevent common signs of ageing from appearing in the first place.

## How do non-ablative lasers work?

Non-ablative lasers penetrate the skin's outer layer, heating the dermis beneath. This heat creates controlled damage that triggers the body's natural healing response. You know the drill – think increased collagen and elastin production for more youthful looking skin. Some non-ablative lasers also target haemoglobin (the red pigment in our blood) and melanin (brown pigment in skin), making them effective in reducing redness and pigmentation.

## THE FACTS

**What to expect**
The therapist will thoroughly cleanse your skin and provide protective goggles to shield your eyes. The laser is then applied to the skin in a controlled manner.

**Does it hurt?**
This can depend on the device but the treatment is not usually painful. In my clinic, for example, we use the Cutera Laser Genesis which feels like laying in hot sun. Other devices may result in mild discomfort.

**Is there any downtime?**
You may notice mild discomfort, temporary redness, and swelling, but these generally subside within a few hours.

**When will I see results?**
Significant results are achieved over multiple sessions (typically between three to six treatments) spaced over several months.

**How long do results last?**
Results can last for between six to twelve months depending on the number of treatments you commit to.

**Recommended brands:** Cutera Laser Genesis, Cutera Erbium Glass, Sciton MOXI, Lynton Motus, Lumenis M22

**Price:** From £600

Some laser treatments may be more affordable (from £100) but you'll need a course of sessions for full results.

# Fractional lasers

If your skin is further along in the aging process, don't worry – there is another type of non-ablative laser that may be suitable for you. Enter fractional lasers.

## How do fractional lasers work?

Fractional lasers focus energy on one small area of the skin at a time, leaving surrounding tissues largely unharmed. The result? Increased collagen regeneration and the production of fresh, healthy skin cells, leading to significant improvements in skin quality and firmness. Fractional lasers are also a great tool for treating fine lines, wrinkles, scars, hyperpigmentation, and skin sagging.

# THE FACTS

**What to expect**
The therapist will thoroughly cleanse your skin and provide protective goggles to shield your eyes. The laser device is then applied to your specific area or areas of concern.

**Does it hurt?**
Fractional laser can be uncomfortable, but they are generally considered tolerable.

**Is there any downtime?**
Downtime can vary from a few days to a week depending on the intensity of the treatment.

**When will I see results?**
You may notice that skin appears brighter and smoother immediately. The full benefits of the treatment are revealed over three months or so.

**How long do results last?**
Results can last between six to eighteen months, depending on the intensity and number of treatments you commit to.

**Recommended brands:** Cutera Erbium Glass (Secret Duo), Fraxel, Sciton Halo, Lynton ResurFace

**Price:** From £500

# Ablative lasers

Ablative lasers are typically used to treat severe skin concerns (such as deep wrinkles, severe sun damage, scarring and significant sagging) and can also be reached for when previous, less aggressive treatments haven't achieved the desired results.

## How do ablative lasers work?

Ablative lasers remove the outer layer of skin (the epidermis) and partially penetrate its underlying layer (the dermis), causing controlled damage. Like non-ablative lasers, they rejuvenate the skin by stimulating the body's natural healing process and promoting the production of collagen and new skin tissue.

Because ablative lasers are more invasive, and carry a higher risk of side effects than non-ablative lasers, these treatments should always be performed by a qualified medical professional.

## Which ablative laser is right for me?

There are two primary types of ablative laser – carbon dioxide and ER:YAG. Here's what you need to know:

### Carbon dioxide ($CO^2$) lasers
When this laser energy is absorbed by the water in skin, the targeted tissue is instantaneously vaporized, removing the outer layers of skin (epidermis) and heating the underlying layer (dermis) to stimulate collagen production.

### Erbium: yttrium-aluminium-garnet (Er:YAG) lasers
Er:YAG lasers are also absorbed by water in the skin but cause less thermal damage to surrounding tissues when compared to $CO^2$ lasers.

This results in a more precise ablation of the skin and fewer unwanted side effects, such as hyperpigmentation.

## THE FACTS

**What to expect**
The practitioner will thoroughly cleanse your skin and provide protective goggles to shield your eyes. The laser device is then moved over the surface of your skin.

**Does it hurt?**
Yes, ablative lasers can be painful, but most find these treatments tolerable. You may notice a stinging sensation that some compare to an elastic band snapping against skin. A topical anaesthetic can be applied to make the treatment more comfortable.

**Is there any downtime?**
Downtime depends on the type of laser used. Er:YAG lasers tend to require just one to two weeks, while $CO_2$ lasers can result in two to three weeks of downtime before you're able to return to normal activities. Side effects include redness, swelling, discomfort and skin weeping or oozing. Diligent aftercare is needed.

**When will I see results?**
As skin heals you'll notice improvements in its texture and tone. The full results become apparent after three to six months.

**How long do results last?**
Results typically last three to five years.

**Recommended brands:** Lumenis UltraPulse $CO_2$, Sciton ProFractional, Lynton SmartXide

**Price:** From £1,000

## A note on darker skin

Ablative laser treatments can be performed on darker skin tones. However, pre-treatment skin preparation is crucial to reduce the risk of post-inflammatory hyperpigmentation.

# Intense pulsed light (IPL)

**BEST FOR:** Reducing signs of sun damage (age spots and pigmentation); tackling broken capillaries; minimising rosacea; supporting general skin rejuvenation.

## How does IPL work?

While thoughts of pulsing light might take you back to your clubbing days, this treatment is something very different! Unlike lasers that emit a single light wavelength, intense pulsed light devices emit a broad spectrum of light across a range of wavelengths.

Specific wavelengths are used to target different skin concerns. If you're hoping to minimise pigmentation, the device will be set to target melanin, for example. If redness, rosacea or spider veins are your primary concern, the device will instead target haemoglobin, the molecule that gives blood its red colour.

When the light energy is absorbed by skin, the heat causes controlled thermal damage that breaks down the pigmented cells or coagulates blood vessels without harming the surrounding tissue. The targeted, damaged tissues are then whisked away by the body's natural healing processes, leading to a clearer and more even complexion.

The thermal effects of IPL can also stimulate collagen and elastin production for improved skin texture, firmness and reduced fine lines and wrinkles over time – a bonus!

## Is IPL right for my skin?

IPL treatments are generally most effective on lighter skin tones. Darker skins face a greater risk of pigmentation as well as burns or skin absorbing too much light. For this reason, it's important to have a thorough skin assessment with a professional before proceeding with treatment.

## THE FACTS

**What to expect**
The therapist will thoroughly cleanse your skin and give your protective eye goggles to wear. The handheld IPL device is then applied to any areas of concern.

**Does it hurt?**
IPL treatments can be a little uncomfortable but are generally tolerable. You may notice a stinging or zapping sensation.

**Is there any downtime?**
When compared to other treatments that target veins or pigmentation, IPL comes with minimal downtime. Areas of pigmentation will usually darken and flake off within one to two weeks. Veins can look like little cat scratches and take up to two weeks to disappear.

**When will I see results?**
Most people need between three and five sessions spaced several

weeks apart for optimal results. You'll notice gradual improvements within one to two weeks of each session.

**How long do results last?**
Results can last between six months to several years depending on the condition of your skin and how diligent you are with sun protection. Periodical maintenance treatments can help to preserve results.

**Recommended brands:** Cutera Limelight, Candela, Cynosure, Sciton BBL, Lumina Dynamix

**Price:** From £150

# Microneedling

**BEST FOR:** Softening fine lines and wrinkles; improving skin texture; minimising scarring and visible pores; tightening skin.

## How does microneedling work?

This therapy involves using a device with tiny needles to make thousands of micro punctures in the skin. These small skin injuries activate a wound-healing response and the production of collagen. New blood vessels also appear to supply oxygen to the stimulated tissue. The end result? Tighter, healthier and more youthful-looking skin.

Microneedling treatments vary depending on how deep the needles go. This can vary from 0.1-1mm (shallow microneedling) all the way up to 3mm (deep microneedling). Microneedling can also be combined with skin-rejuvenating ingredients, such as exosomes (see page 136) or peptides, which are absorbed into the deeper layers of skin thanks to the microinjuries. This is often described as a MesoFacial.

## THE FACTS

**What to expect**
The therapist will thoroughly cleanse your skin before applying the microneedling device to a the targeted area of concern.

**Does it hurt?**
Yes, microneedling treatments can be uncomfortable and an anaesthetic cream is required. Shallow microneedling treatments are more comfortable than deeper ones.

**Is there any downtime?**
You may notice pinprick marks and skin redness but there is minimal downtime – particularly after shallow microneedling. Deeper needling treatments may require two to four days downtime.

**When will I see results?**
You may see improvements in skin after a few weeks, but the full results are revealed after several months as your skin produces new collagen, elastin and hyaluronic acid. Most people need multiple treatments spaced several weeks apart.

**How long do results last?**
Results last for between several months to a year, depending on the depth of needling and number of treatments you commit to. Periodical maintenance treatments can help to preserve results.

**Recommended brands:** DermaPen 4, Rejuvapen

**Price:** From £200

> ### Don't try this at home
>
> You may have come across at-home microneedling devices, such as a derma roller, that target the skin's most superficial layer (the epidermis). Professional devices, by contrast, are designed to penetrate deeper into the skin (the dermis). This delivers better results but must only be used in a clinical setting with sterile, single-use needles.

# Exosomes

**BEST FOR:** Improving skin tone and texture; reducing pigmentation; smoothing lines and wrinkles; minimising dark under-eye circles, scarring and visible pores; calming rosacea and redness; repairing the skin barrier.

## How do exosomes work?

While technically not a technology, exosomes are a powerful, regenerative ingredient causing a buzz in the world of aesthetics. They can be paired with treatments such as microneedling, fractional laser and radiofrequency to improve results, and heal and support skin from the inside out.

Exosomes are tiny, naturally-occurring bubbles (the technical word is vesicles) that are released by our cells. They play an essential role in the body's healing processes and support cell communication, carrying proteins, fats and genetic material from one cell to another.

They've been ignored by skin scientists for many years who have only recently begun to wake up to how successfully they promote skin regeneration and healing, while slowing down ageing processes.

Studies now show that they can stimulate our fibroblasts to produce more collagen and boost our supply of hyaluronic acid and essential fats for better moisture retention and plumper-looking skin. Research also shows these powerhouses accelerate wound healing and soothe inflammation, redness and irritation.

# THE FACTS

**What to expect**
The therapist will thoroughly cleanse your skin before applying an exosome serum. They will then follow up with the partner treatment – whether that be microneedling, laser or radio frequency. In my clinic, I prefer to pair exosomes with microneedling and a device called Target Cool. This uses nitrous oxide to further propel exosomes into skin.

**Does it hurt?**
This depends on which treatment exosomes are paired with.

**Is there any downtime?**
This depends on which treatment exosomes are paired with, but exosomes can help to speed up skin healing and reduce downtime.

**When will I see results?**
Results last for between several months to a year, depending on which treatment exosomes are paired with.

**How long do results last?**
You may see improvements in skin after a few weeks, but the full results are revealed after several months as your skin regenerates and produces new collagen, elastin and hyaluronic acid.

**Recommended brands:** E50 Exosomes

**Price:** From £400

# Platelet-rich plasma therapy (PRP)

**BEST FOR:** Reducing fine lines and wrinkles; improving skin texture; minimising dark under eye circles; tightening skin; correcting sun damage.

## How does PRP work?

PRP therapy (also known as 'the vampire facial') involves injecting plasma that's been extracted from your own blood to areas in need of rejuvenation – whether that be the face, hands or neck. This plasma is packed with platelets and growth factors that help to identify and repair skin damage. It sounds like something out of a scary movie but hear me out! For those who want to avoid injecting foreign substances (such as toxin or fillers), PRP offers a natural alternative.

# THE FACTS

**What to expect**
First, a small amount of blood (about 15 ml) is taken from your arm. The plasma is then extracted from the blood (by whizzing it in a centrifuge) and injected into your skin.

**Does it hurt?**
No, PRP shouldn't hurt.

**Is there any downtime?**
You may notice small pinpricks on skin where the plasma has been injected but there is no downtime. And, as PRP uses your own blood, the risk of infection or an allergic reaction is minimal.

**When will I see results?**
You'll notice improvements over a period of weeks to months. For best results, commit to a course of treatments every four to six weeks.

**How long do results last?**
Results last between twelve to eighteen months, depending on your skin's condition and the number of treatments you commit to. Periodical maintenance treatments can help to preserve results.

**Price:** From £300

# Fat-busting treatments

**BEST FOR:** Minimising a double chin; improving the contour of the neck.

Both lipolysis injections and 'fat freezing' treatments can be used to tackle areas of unwanted fat – particularly fat that gathers under the chin. Here's what you need to know:

## Lipolysis injections

### How do lipolysis injections work?

Lipolysis injections contain deoxycholic acid, which ruptures fat cell membranes. Once ruptured, this unwanted fat is absorbed by the body and disposed of. These injections are particularly effective because, once the fat cells are destroyed, they do not regrow. However, it's important to maintain a stable weight after treatment to prevent new fat deposits from forming in their place.

### THE FACTS

**What to expect**
First, your practitioner (usually a medical professional) will apply a topical anaesthetic or ice pack to numb the area and minimise

discomfort. Multiple small injections of deoxycholic acid are then administered directly into the fat layer.

### Does it hurt?
You may experience a stinging sensation, but this treatment shouldn't be painful.

### Is there any downtime?
Common side effects including swelling, bruising, pain or redness, at the injection site – although these typically subside within a few days to weeks. Clients can usually resume normal activities shortly after the procedure.

### When will I see results?
Results are usually seen after two to four treatment sessions, spaced about four to six weeks apart.

### How long do results last?
The results can be permanent if your overall weight remains stable.

**Recommended brands:** Aqualyx

**Price:** From £250

## Cryolipolysis (fat freezing)

### How does fat freezing work?

This treatment has one of my favourite origin stories: it was developed after two America doctors noticed that children who frequently sucked on ice lollies had indentations in their cheek fat! Understandably curious, they investigated further, and their findings led to the creation of fat freezing treatments.

During this treatment, fat cells start to slowly die when exposed to temperatures below 4°C. Once dead, they are gradually eliminated by the body.

Cryolipolysis is particularly appealing as it's non-invasive (unlike liposuction) and results in the permanent removal of targeted fat cells. Once the fat cells are gone, they're gone for good!

## THE FACTS

**What to expect**
Your therapist will place a small, rectangular bucket-shaped treatment device onto the skin. A gel pad is applied to the skin as a protective layer to prevent it from adhering to the device. The device then suctions in a section of fat (a bit like a plunger) and cools it to 4°C or lower. After the cooling process is complete, the near-frozen lump of fat is gently massaged back into shape. The procedure is repeated as necessary, with the device being applied to different sections of skin and fat.

**Does it hurt?**
The treatment shouldn't hurt but you may notice a tingling, stinging or aching sensation as fat is frozen.

**Is there any downtime?**
Skin may appear red or swollen but this should clear up in one to two days.

**When will I see results?**
Cryolipolysis is not an instant fix. The body's natural process of breaking down and flushing out fat deposits can take between three to six months.

**How long do results last?**
The results can be permanent if your overall weight remains stable.

**Recommended brands:** Coolsculpting

**Price:** From £500

---

### Fat-freezing risks

While cryolipolysis is considered a safe and effective treatment, it's not without its risks. Research shows that common side effects include erythema (skin redness), swelling, and pain – all mild and transient. The more worrying side effect is paradoxical adipose hyperplasia in which – 'paradoxically' – fat piles onto the treatment area instead of disappearing. This is very rare but recently hit headlines after Linda Evangelista was left, in her words, 'permanently deformed' by her fat-freezing treatment. These headlines are scary, but the evidence shows that this treatment is, in the vast majority of cases, a safe and effective alternative to surgical intervention.

# Wet microdermabrasion (HydraFacial)

**BEST FOR:** Deep cleansing; minimising visible pores; reducing puffiness; increasing skin radiance and hydration.

## How does wet microdermabrasion work?

The perfect pick-me-up for those with busy schedules, wet microdermabrasion (better known by the brand name – HydraFacial) combines multiple techniques to deeply hydrate, cleanse and exfoliate skin for a clearer and more radiant complexion.

## THE FACTS

**What to expect**
A HydraFacial has five or six distinct steps:

1. **Lymphatic drainage massage**
   Your therapist will first perform lymphatic drainage to enhance circulation, reduce puffiness, help to eliminate toxins and promote overall skin health.

2. **Cleanse and peel**
   Next, they'll draw a wand with an attached exfoliating tip across

the face. The tip is infused with a gentle peeling solution to exfoliate the skin and remove dead skin cells.

3. **Extraction**
   Using a gentle suction device, debris and impurities are painlessly removed from pores to clear congestion and reduce the likelihood of breakouts.

4. **Hydration**
   Once again using the wand (but with a different special tip), nourishing moisturisers, antioxidants, and peptides are applied to the skin for intense hydration and protection.

5. **Skin boosters**
   If desired, specially formulated serums can also be used to target specific skin concerns – including fine lines, wrinkles, acne, mild hyperpigmentation and sun damage.

6. **LED light therapy**
   The treatment concludes with red and blue LED therapy to support skin healing and health. The red light reduces redness and stimulates collagen production, while blue light targets bacteria to help prevent future breakouts.

**Does it hurt?**
No – most find the HydraFacial an enjoyable and relaxing experience.

**Is there any downtime?**
No

**When will I see results?**
There's no waiting around involved with a HydraFacial: this treatment offers immediate results in terms of improved skin texture and radiance.

**How long do results last?**
Results typically last two to four weeks.

**Recommended brands:** HydraFacial (avoid cheap copies such as HydroFacial)

**Price:** From £100

# Injectable skin-boosters

**BEST FOR:** Minimising visible pores, redness, crepiness, dark under-eye circles and wrinkles; improving skin tone and elasticity; increasing skin radiance; tightening skin.

We're seeing an uplift in the popularity of injectable skin-boosting treatments at my MediSpa, and it's easy to see why: these injectables require minimal downtime and deliver speedy results. Injectable skin-boosters are also cost effective and can amplify the results of energy-based treatments such as radiofrequency, ultrasound and lasers. There are two key injectable ingredients to look out for – polynucleotides and hyaluronic acid.

## Polynucleotide (PN) injections

**BEST FOR:** Minimising visible pores, crepiness, sun damage, pigmentation, fine lines and wrinkles; hydrating skin; improving skin tone and elasticity.

### How do PN injections work?

Nucleotides are the star ingredient in PN injections. These are the building blocks that make up DNA and RNA – an essential molecule involved in healthy gene and cell function. When we inject nucleotides, this helpful ingredient gets to work regenerating and repairing skin from the inside out. We see fresh collagen and elastin production, for enhanced elasticity and skin firmness, as well as improved hydration and a noticeable reduction in skin inflammation. This skin-soothing effect further minimises signs of skin ageing and sun damage.

# Hyaluronic acid injections (injectable moisturisers)

**BEST FOR:** Hydrating and plumping skin; improving skin tone and elasticity; increasing skin radiance.

### How do HA injections work?

HA injections have a dual action: they hydrate skin from the inside-out while also triggering bio-stimulation. This process encourages the skin to regenerate itself and produce more supportive collagen and elastin for pro-ageing benefits.

## THE FACTS

**What to expect**
The therapist will thoroughly cleanse your skin before injecting your ingredient of choice into multiple areas of face, neck or hands.

**Does it hurt?**
Injections aren't pleasant (expect a short, sharp sting) but shouldn't be painful. In some cases, anaesthetic can be applied to reduce discomfort.

**Is there any downtime?**
As with any injectable procedure, there is a small risk of bruising that can take a few days to disappear. But, in most cases, there is no downtime – skin may look a little red or show signs of small pinprick injection marks, but these subside within a few hours of the treatment.

**When will I see results?**
You'll notice improvements within a few weeks. For optimal results, two to three sessions are required, each spaced one month apart.

**How long do results last?**
Results can last between six to twelve months depending on your skin's condition and the number of treatments you commit to.

**Recommended brands:**
PN injections: Philart, Ameela, Plinest
HA injections: Profhilo, SuneKos, Hal75, Jalupro

**Price:** From £250

# Toxin injections

**BEST FOR:** Reducing lines and wrinkles; lifting brows or jowls; softening neck bands.

## How do toxin injections work?

Toxin injections (better known by the brand name – Botox) remain one of the most popular and best known non-surgical treatments. This is thanks to their remarkable ability to smooth wrinkles and create a lifting effect. While originally approved for medical conditions such as blepharospasm (eye spasms) and strabismus (crossed eyes), these injections have since gone on to revolutionise cosmetic treatments worldwide.

The active ingredient is a purified form of botulinum toxin that, when injected in small doses, temporarily paralyses muscles. Our faces move less and this smooths and prevents fine lines and wrinkles.

While toxin injections are best known for tackling fine lines and wrinkles, they can do a whole lot more! When injected into the depressor muscles of the face, for example, they can counteract their downward pull, leading to a lifted and fresh-faced appearance. We can also use toxin injections to lift the brow and relax the muscles that pull the corners of our mouth downwards.

Other common uses for toxin injections include:

- Treating the 'eleven' lines between eyebrows
- Reducing crow's feet (the wrinkles at the sides of the eyes)
- Softening horizontal lines on the forehead
- Minimising 'bunny lines' (the horizontal wrinkles at the top of the nose)
- Reducing muscle clenching in the jaw by targeting the masseter, the main chewing muscle
- Softening a stringy-looking neck to make it appear longer and slimmer

### All in the dose

It's important to choose an experienced and skilful practitioner when booking toxin injections as the technique and dose can make or break your final outcome.

A well-trained practitioner will consider your facial anatomy, the size of the muscle, the extent of muscle activity, and your desired aesthetic outcomes. They'll also think about how facial muscles interact to ensure no 'supporting' muscles are accidentally relaxed – this can result in unwanted facial expressions, drooping or an asymmetrical appearance.

> ## Is Botox safe?
>
> The idea of injecting a toxin into your body may sound scary. However, there's a large body of evidence that shows toxin injections are safe and effective when administered by a qualified professional. As with any medical procedure, they come with potential risks and side effects. These can include temporary bruising, swelling, redness, or tenderness at the injection site. In rare cases, patients may experience headaches, drooping eyelids, or allergic reactions.

## THE FACTS

**What to expect**
A practitioner will thoroughly cleanse your skin before injecting a small amount of toxin to the targeted muscles.

**Does it hurt?**
Injections aren't pleasant (expect a short, sharp sting) but shouldn't be painful.

**Is there any downtime?**
As with any injectable procedure, there is a small risk of bruising with can take a few days to disappear. But, in most cases, there's no downtime. You may notice small pinprick injection marks, but these subside within a few hours of the treatment.

**When will I see results?**
Full results are usually visible after ten to fourteen days.

**How long do results last?**
Results typically last between three to four months.

**Recommended brands:** Botox, Bocouture, Azzalure

**Price:** From £200

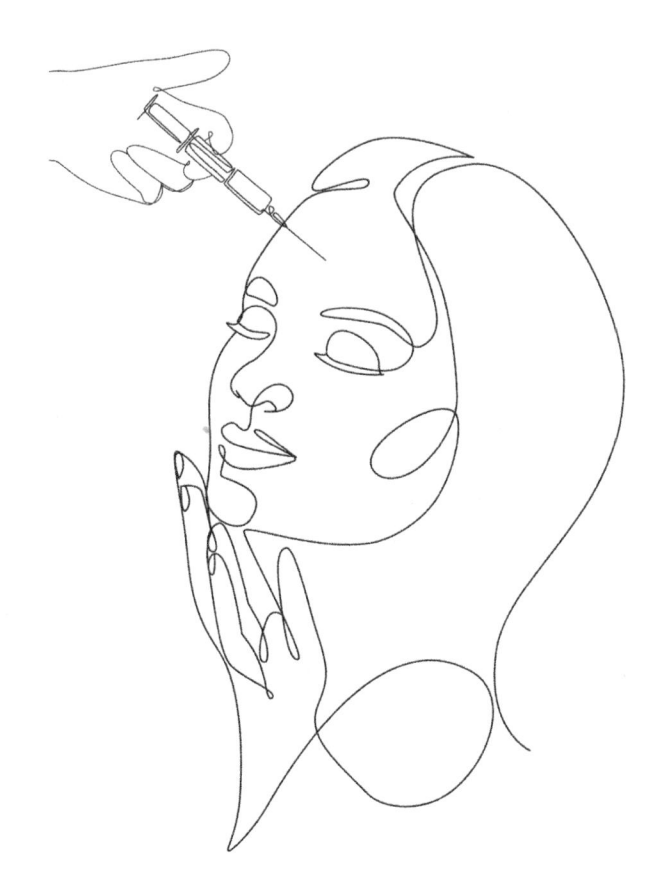

# Fillers

**BEST FOR:** Adding volume; enhancing the shape of the face; softening lines, wrinkles and folds.

I think it's unfortunate that fillers have gained a bad reputation in recent years. It's true that they can create an exaggerated, cartoon-like appearance when overused – particularly in younger individuals who don't need them. But, when used in moderation and applied skilfully, fillers can deliver fabulous results.

## How do fillers work?

Dermal fillers are gels made of high-density ingredients that are injected into skin to provide structure and support. When fillers first came to market, they were used to smooth specific 'stand out' lines and wrinkles (such as the lines that run from the nose to the corners of the mouth). Nowadays, they are used more holistically to make subtle adjustments to the shape and structure of the face. They can help add volume and contour to areas that have lost definition due to ageing and bone resorption. The cheeks are another popular treatment area, as is the jawline and chin. I've recently added a touch of filler to my own for improved definition.

## Which filler is right for me?

Not all filler is created equal. There are three key types to look out for: hyaluronic acid filler, calcium hydroxylapatite filler and poly-l-lactic acid filler. Here's what you need to know:

# Hyaluronic acid (HA)

**BEST FOR:** Adding volume to lips and cheeks; minimising fine lines and wrinkles; correcting under-eye shadows.

THE PROS:
A powerful moisturiser, HA is often used in dermal fillers as it naturally occurs in the human body and is easy to reverse. As such, it's ideal for those seeking temporary adjustments or who are apprehensive about permanent cosmetic procedures.

THE CONS:
HA filler is less long lasting than other dermal fillers. It can also encourage fluid retention which is not ideal when treating complaints such as under-eye bags. While HA fillers are technically dissolvable, they're still long-lasting. MRI scans taken 15 years after injections have found HA still within the skin.

**Recommended brands:** Juvederm, Restylane®

---

# Calcium hydroxylapatite (CaHA) filler

**BEST FOR:** Minimising deep wrinkles; enhancing bone structure (cheekbones and jawline); tightening and regenerating skin.

THE PROS:
CaHA is thick, sticky and viscous, making it the perfect choice for addressing deeper wrinkles and enhancing bone structure (such as cheekbones). CaHA also promotes tissue regeneration which means it can help to soften severe facial wrinkles and folds (for long-lasting results) while it fills them in.

THE CONS:
CaHA injections can sometimes create nodules or lumps under the skin, which may require treatment or surgical removal. Unlike HA filler, CaHA cannot easily be dissolved, making it more difficult to reverse or make corrections if we're unhappy with the result. These fillers are longer lasting than other fillers, but still require periodical touch-ups.

**Recommended brands:** Radiesse®

## Poly-L-lactic acid (PLLA) fillers

**BEST FOR:** Restoring natural-looking volume; improving collagen production; smoothing fine lines; long-lasting facial rejuvenation.

THE PROS:
PLLA is a multi-tasking filler that stimulates our natural collagen production while restoring volume. This leads to lasting improvements in the texture and volume of skin. In fact, PLLA fillers are more long-lasting than HA filler, with results still visible after two years.

THE CONS:
PLLA fillers don't deliver immediate results – it takes several treatments over a few months to see the full results as collagen production ramps up. This treatment comes with a higher risk of developing small bumps under skin that may require treatment or surgical removal. The injection technique can also be trickier, so hunting down a skilled and experienced injector is even more important.

**Recommended brands:** Sculptra®, Silhouette Soft®

## Are fillers safe?

Fillers are safe and effective but there are some notable (if rare) side effects. These include allergic reactions, infection at the site of injection and – most concerning – tissue necrosis. Tissue necrosis is a rare but serious complication that occurs when filler blocks a blood vessel, cutting off blood supply to the surrounding tissue. Without blood, this tissue dies: the first signs are pain and whitening of the skin, which later progresses into darkening skin, blisters, and ulcers. In these rare cases, speedy intervention from a medic is vital to minimise tissue damage and ensure the best outcome.

This is why I don't recommend getting filler injected by a non-medic. I'm sure there are therapists out there who are highly skilled and very capable, but the risk of side effects makes it much safer to have a doctor or nurse on hand.

Look for a skilled practitioner who has in-depth knowledge of facial anatomy, has attended advanced cadaver courses, has at least five years of experience and has (preferably) been recommended to you by someone you know. Take time to look at samples of their work to ensure their style matches your desired aesthetic outcome.

In cases of necrosis, hyaluronidase can be used to dissolve HA fillers to restore blood flow (when an HA-based filler is used), while topical nitroglycerin may help by dilating blood vessels and improving blood flow. Taking Asprin can also help as it increases blood flow to the area.

# THE FACTS

**What to expect**
A practitioner will thoroughly cleanse your skin before injecting filler to the desired area.

**Does it hurt?**
Injections aren't pleasant (expect a short, sharp sting) but shouldn't be painful.

**Is there any downtime?**
Minimal downtime is required. You may notice slight swelling in the area which disappears after a day or two. If filler has been applied to lips, swelling can take one to two weeks to settle. As with any injectable, there's a risk of bruising which can take longer to disappear entirely.

**When will I see results?**
Results are immediate.

**How long do results last?**
One to three years, depending on the type of filler.

**Recommended brands**
See on previous pages.

**Price:** From £200

# LED light therapy

**BEST FOR:** Reducing fine lines and wrinkles; minimising pigmentation; improving rosacea and redness; enhancing overall skin texture.

## How does LED light therapy work?

This non-invasive therapy has become increasingly popular as it's extremely safe and comfortable. Who wouldn't want to rest under a canopy of skin-transforming lights?

During a LED therapy treatment, the small LED bulbs emit light at different wavelengths and colours that penetrate the skin and deliver different skin benefits. Red light, for example, stimulates fibroblasts (the cells responsible for producing collagen) for smoother and more rejuvenated skin. Red light can also help to soothe inflammation and redness, creating a more even skin tone. This is particularly beneficial for those with rosacea.

Blue and yellow lights are also commonly used during LED treatments. Blue light has been shown to enhance skin hydration levels by improving barrier function. The result? A healthier and more radiant appearance.

Meanwhile, yellow light therapies can help to reduce pigmentation and improve skin elasticity. This makes yellow light (and not sunshine) the ideal choice for those with sun-damaged skin.

Using a combination of different wavelengths and colours can also be effective. The pairing of red and near-infrared LEDs, for instance, has been shown to rejuvenate skin by stimulating both collagen and elastin production, for improved skin texture and elasticity, as well as wrinkle reduction.

LED light therapy can be used as a standalone treatment or as a healing addition to more intensive therapies such as microneedling, fractional radio frequency, or skin peels.

## THE FACTS

**What to expect**
A therapist will thoroughly cleanse your skin before giving you a pair of protective goggles. You'll then rest under a panel of LED lights for approximately 30-45 minutes.

**Does it hurt?**
Not at all. This is a painless, relaxing treatment.

**Is there any downtime?**
There's no downtime after LED therapy. In fact, skin may look calmer and happier after treatment.

**When will I see results?**
You may notice an immediate improvement in skin hydration and radiance. It can take several months of regular treatments to see improvements in fine lines, wrinkles, skin elasticity and pigmentation.

**How long do results last?**
Results can last for several months depending on your skin's condition and the number of treatments you commit to. Periodical maintenance treatments can help to preserve results.

**Recommended brands:** Dermalux, Omnilux

**Price:** From £40

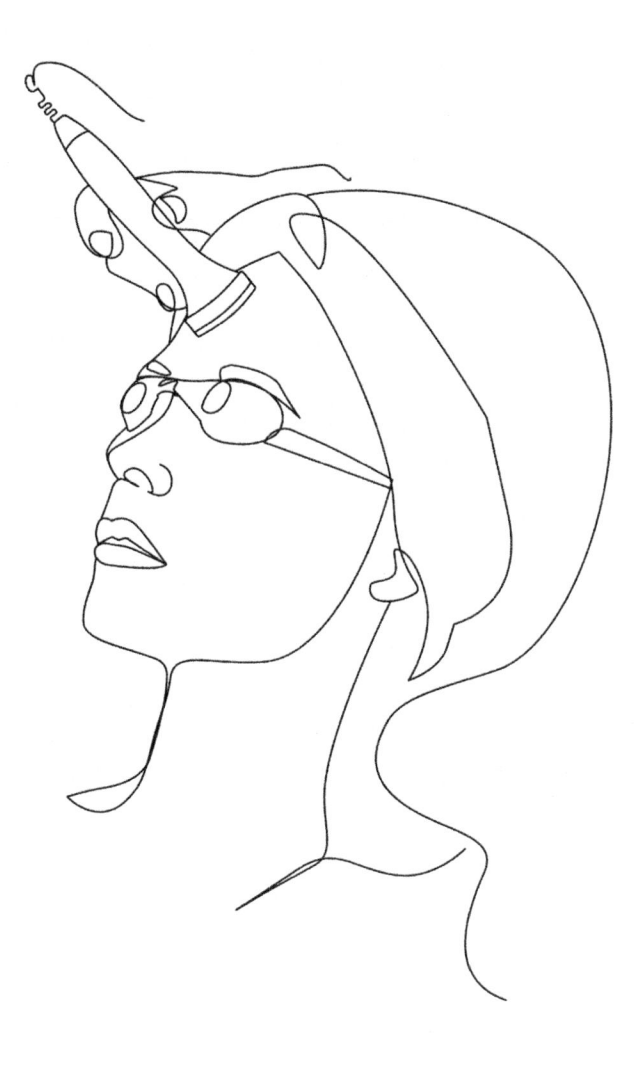

# Facial thread lifts

**BEST FOR:** Lifting sagging skin; stimulating collagen and elastin production.

## How do facial thread lifts work?

Gone are the days of going under the knife for our face lift. A facial thread lift is a minimally invasive procedure designed to light and tighten sagging skin without the risks and downtime associated with surgery. The lift is achieved by threading a biodegradable material into the fat that sits below skin. This thread is then pulled right to hoist and lift any areas of sagging. Over time, the biodegradable thread dissolves but, in many cases, it works to stimulate collagen production to take its place – creating more long-lasting results.

## Which facial thread lift is right for me?

There are several types of threads used in these non-invasive lifts, each with their own pros and cons.

## Polydioxanone (PDO) threads

These threads are made from a biodegradable material that dissolves naturally over time. They come in three textures – smooth, twisted, or barbed.

While all three can encourage collagen production, they also each have individual benefits. Smooth threads tend to be used for skin-rejuvenation; twisted threads provide more volume in depleted areas; and barbed threads are used for more significant lifting.

PDO threads typically dissolve within six months, but the collagen that builds around them helps maintain the treatment's effects for a few more months.

## Poly-L-lactic acid (PLLA) threads

PLLA threads are also biodegradable but last longer than PDO threads and often come with cones or barbs that anchor into tissue for a more dramatic lift. They also work to stimulate collagen production for more durable results.

These threads gradually dissolve over twelve to eighteen months, with the lifting effect lasting up to two years or more (thanks to collagen production).

## Polycaprolactone (PCL) threads

The longest lasting of the three biodegradable materials, PCL threads are particularly effective for achieving durable skin tightening and a noticeable lift.

They take about two years to dissolve, with the cosmetic effects lasting even longer due to prolonged collagen synthesis.

## Are facial thread lifts safe?

This treatment carries fewer risks than a surgical face lift but there are still a few key adverse effects to be aware of:

**Infection:** any treatment that breaks the surface of skin carries a risk of infection.

**Asymmetry:** If threads are not placed with care, it's possible to end up with a lopsided appearance where one side of the face looks different to the other.

**Nerve damage:** Incorrect placement of facial threads can damage facial nerves leading to temporary or, in rare cases, permanent facial paralysis.

As with any treatment, a successful outcome depends on the skill and experience of the practitioner performing the treatment. I've seen many clients who have not been happy with the outcome of their thread lifts so I wouldn't recommend this treatment unless you're confident you have found a skilled practitioner who comes highly recommended.

# THE FACTS

**What to expect**
A practitioner will thoroughly cleanse skin before applying a local anaesthetic. Next, a fine needle or cannula is used to insert threads into the fat layer below skin. Finally, the threads are anchored into place and gently tightened to provide a lift.

**Does it hurt?**
You shouldn't feel anything during the treatment thanks to the local anaesthetic.

**Is there any downtime?**
You may notice some swelling or bruising but this should disappear within a week of the treatment.

**When will I see results?**
You'll notice immediate improvements, but the full results will be evident after two to three weeks.

**How long do results last?**
Between six months to several years, depending on the type of thread (see above).

**Recommended brands:** Silhouette Soft®, Silhouette InstaLift™ Threads
**Price:** From £1,500

# Permanent makeup

**BEST FOR:** Enhancing features that fade as we age.

As we get older, our eyes, lips and brows can lose their shape and prominence. Our once bold lashes lose their thickness, our brows gradually thin, and our lips appear smaller – these changes compound to create an overall impression of fading features.

Permanent makeup is a great non-invasive solution that can trick the eye and restore volume and vibrancy to our features. As a permanent makeup artist with over twenty-five years' experience, I've seen first-hand just how transformative this treatment can be.

## How does permanent makeup work?

Permanent makeup, also known as micropigmentation, does exactly what it says on the tin. It can enhance your features in the same way makeup can but lasts much longer – so no more daily hassle of reapplying traditional cosmetics. By embedding medical-grade mineral pigments into the deeper layers of the skin, a skilled permanent makeup artist can simulate the appearance of fuller brows, thicker lashes, and more defined, fuller lips.

## Which treatment is right for me?

A skilled permanent makeup artists can enhance your features in a number of ways.

## Brows

Permanent brows can be created with hair strokes, a powdered effect, or a blend of both.

The technician will start by using a pencil to carefully draw on brows in a way that complements your face shape and brow bone. In some cases, if the natural brow slopes downwards (making the eye area droop), the outer half of the brows can be repositioned to create a more youthful, lifted appearance. Sometimes, this simple technique can make you look 10 years younger!

Once the shape is decided, a pigment blend is mixed to match to existing brow hair and chosen to complement your eyes, skin tone, and hair colour. This is then placed into the deeper layers of the skin, simulating the appearance of hair strokes. I prefer a microblading tool which allows for crisper, cleaner hair strokes. The vibration of the permanent makeup needle can sometimes result in more blurred, fuzzy-edged hair strokes.

## Eyes

If eyes are losing their definition, placing a fine line of pigment through the lash line can cheat thicker, more defined lashes. Different needles can be used to achieve different looks – from a defined 'eyeliner' look to a softer and more subtle effect.

## Lips

If lip filler isn't for you, permanent makeup can help enhance lip fullness and symmetry. The technician will mix a pigment to match your natural lip colour or a 'your lips but better' colour. They'll sketch the new lip shape with a lip liner first before using a fine needle to tattoo it into place. A softer needle is then used to blend the colour evenly across the lips.

---

### Find a skilled technician

When selecting a permanent makeup artist, look for someone who has at least five years' experience, whose work you have seen, and who comes highly recommended. Reading Google reviews can also be helpful.

Avoid technicians offering suspiciously low prices, as this often indicates subpar service. I would also be cautious of overly edited images on social media offering unrealistic results.

A reputable technician will provide a pre-treatment consultation to discuss your needs and conduct a skin test. A follow-up appointment should also be included in the cost to allow for any necessary touch-ups.

# THE FACTS

**What to expect**
The treatment can vary depending on which area of the face is being treated (see details on previous page).

**Does it hurt?**
Clients are often concerned that the treatment will be painful. However, an experienced technician will be able to keep discomfort to a minimum through the correct use of topical anaesthetics.

**Is there any downtime?**
It can take up to a week for skin to heal. During this time, the surface pigment is exfoliated away, revealing the healed colour underneath. If pigment has been applied to eyes you may notice swelling for up to two days but you're fine to go about your business.

**When will I see results?**
After one week.

**How long do results last?**
Results last between one and three years.

**Recommended brands:** KB Pro, Tina Davies

**Price:** From £200

# References

Cleveland Clinic. (2021). Cortisol.
https://my.clevelandclinic.org/health/articles/22187-cortisol

Cleveland Clinic. (2022). Endorphins. Available from:
https://my.clevelandclinic.org/health/body/23040-endorphins

Mayo Clinic. (2023). Positive thinking: Stop negative self-talk to reduce stress.
https://www.mayoclinic.org/healthy-lifestyle/stress-management/in-depth/positive-thinking/art-20043950

Giltay, E.J., et al. (2007). Lifestyle and dietary correlates of dispositional optimism in men: The Zutphen Elderly Study. Available from:
https://pubmed.ncbi.nlm.nih.gov/17980220/

The Skin Cancer Foundation. (2021).
UV radiation & your skin. Available from:
https://www.skincancer.org/risk-factors/uv-radiation/

Reilly, D.M., and Lozano, J. (2021). Skin collagen through the lifestages: importance for skin health and beauty. Available from:
https://www.oaepublish.com/articles/2347-9264.2020.153

Mendelson, B., and Wong, C.H. (2012). Changes in the facial skeleton with aging: implications and clinical applications in facial rejuvenation. Available from:
https://pubmed.ncbi.nlm.nih.gov/22580543/

Thornton, M.J. (2013). Estrogens and aging skin. Available from: https://pubmed.ncbi.nlm.nih.gov/24194966/

Stevenson, J., and medical advisory council of the British Menopause Society. (2023). Prevention and treatment of osteoporosis in women. Available from: https://thebms.org.uk/wp-content/uploads/2023/10/06-BMS-ConsensusStatement-Prevention-and-treatment-of-osteoporosis-in-women-SEPT2023-A.pdf

Sator, P.-G., et al. (2001). The influence of hormone replacement therapy on skin ageing. A pilot study. Available from: https://pubmed.ncbi.nlm.nih.gov/11451620/

Gao T, Wang X, Li Y, Ren F. The Role of Probiotics in Skin Health and Related Gut–Skin Axis: A Review. Available from: https://pubmed.ncbi.nlm.nih.gov/37513540/

Boyajian JL, Ghebretatios M, Schaly S, Islam P, Prakash S. Microbiome and Human Aging: Probiotic and Prebiotic Potentials in Longevity, Skin Health and Cellular Senescence. Available from: https://pmc.ncbi.nlm.nih.gov/articles/PMC8705837/

Garcia-Bonete, M.J., Rajan, A., Suriano, F., and Layunta, E. (2023). The Underrated Gut Microbiota Helminths, Bacteriophages, Fungi, and Archaea. Available from: https://pubmed.ncbi.nlm.nih.gov/37629622/

Valdes, A.M., Walter, J., Segal, E., and Spector, T.D. (2018). Role of the gut microbiota in nutrition and health. Available from: https://www.bmj.com/content/361/bmj.k2179

Al Bander, Z., Nitert, M.D., Mousa, A., and Naderpoor, N. (2020). The Gut Microbiota and Inflammation: An Overview. Available from: https://pubmed.ncbi.nlm.nih.gov/33086688/

Pickett, K., et al. (2015). Educational interventions to improve quality of life in people with chronic inflammatory skin diseases: systematic reviews of clinical effectiveness and cost-effectiveness. Available from: https://www.ncbi.nlm.nih.gov/books/NBK321885/

Krajmalnik-Brown, R., Ilhan, Z.E., Kang, D.W., and DiBaise, J.K. (2012). Effects of gut microbes on nutrient absorption and energy regulation. Available from: https://pubmed.ncbi.nlm.nih.gov/22367888/

Woo, Y.R., and Kim, H.S. (2024). Interaction between the microbiota and the skin barrier in aging skin: a comprehensive review. Available from: https://pubmed.ncbi.nlm.nih.gov/38312314/

Qi, X., Yun, C., Pang, Y., and Qiao, J. (2021). The impact of the gut microbiota on the reproductive and metabolic endocrine system. Available from: https://www.ncbi.nlm.nih.gov/pmc/articles/PMC7971312/

Yano, J.M., et al. (2015). Indigenous Bacteria from the Gut Microbiota Regulate Host Serotonin Biosynthesis. Available from https://pubmed.ncbi.nlm.nih.gov/25860609/

Fu, J., Zheng, Y., Gao, Y., and Xu, W. (2022). Dietary Fiber Intake and Gut Microbiota in Human Health. Microorganisms. Available from: https://www.ncbi.nlm.nih.gov/pmc/articles/PMC9787832/

British Dietetic Association. (n.d.). Probiotics and gut health. Available from: https://www.bda.uk.com/resource/probiotics.html

Shi, Z. (2019). Gut Microbiota: An Important Link between Western Diet and Chronic Diseases. Available from: https://www.ncbi.nlm.nih.gov/pmc/articles/PMC6835660/
Merra, G., Noce, A., Marrone, G., Cintoni, M., Tarsitano, M.G.,

Capacci, A., and De Lorenzo, A. (2020). Influence of Mediterranean Diet on Human Gut Microbiota.
Available from: https://pubmed.ncbi.nlm.nih.gov/33375042/

Mithul Aravind, S., Wichienchot, S., Tsao, R., Ramakrishnan, S., and Chakkaravarthi, S. (2021). Role of dietary polyphenols on gut microbiota, their metabolites and health benefits.
Available from: https://www.sciencedirect.com/science/article/abs/pii/S0963996921000880

Bishehsari, F., et al. (2017). Alcohol and Gut-Derived Inflammation.
Available from: https://www.ncbi.nlm.nih.gov/pmc/articles/PMC5513683/

Palma, L., Marques, L., Buján, J., & Rodrigues, L. (2015). Dietary water affects human skin hydration and biomechanics. Available from: https://pmc.ncbi.nlm.nih.gov/articles/PMC4529263/

Park, S., Kang, S., & Lee, W. (2021). Menopause, Ultraviolet Exposure, and Low Water Intake Potentially Interact with the Genetic Variants Related to Collagen Metabolism Involved in Skin Wrinkle Risk in Middle-Aged Women. Available from:
https://pubmed.ncbi.nlm.nih.gov/33669802/

Seol, J.E., et al. (2024). Effect of Amount of Daily Water Intake and Use of Moisturizer on Skin Barrier Function in Healthy Female Participants.
Available from:
https://www.ncbi.nlm.nih.gov/pmc/articles/PMC11148315/

Killer, S.C., et al. (2014). No Evidence of Dehydration with Moderate Daily Coffee Intake: A Counterbalanced Cross-Over Study in a Free-Living Population. Available from:
https://pubmed.ncbi.nlm.nih.gov/24416202/

Umbayev, B., et al. (2020). Galactose-Induced Skin Aging: The Role of Oxidative Stress. Oxidative Medicine and Cellular Activity. Available from: https://pmc.ncbi.nlm.nih.gov/articles/PMC7317321/

Danby, F.W. (2010). Nutrition and aging skin: sugar and glycation. Available from: https://pubmed.ncbi.nlm.nih.gov/20620757/

Brown, M.J. (2019). What Are Advanced Glycation End Products (AGEs). Available from: https://www.healthline.com/nutrition/advanced-glycation-end-products

Ma, X., et al. (2022). Excessive intake of sugar: An accomplice of inflammation. Available from: https://www.ncbi.nlm.nih.gov/pmc/articles/PMC9471313/

Pickett K, Loveman E, Kalita N, et al. Educational interventions to improve quality of life in people with chronic inflammatory skin diseases: systematic reviews of clinical effectiveness and cost-effectiveness. Available from: https://www.ncbi.nlm.nih.gov/books/NBK321885/

Danby, F.W. (2010). Nutrition and aging skin: sugar and glycation. Available from: https://pubmed.ncbi.nlm.nih.gov/20620757/

Haye, V. (2023). Alcohol and urination: what is the link? Available from: https://www.medicalnewstoday.com/articles/why-does-alcohol-make-you-pee

House of Commons Library (2021), 'Alcohol statistics: England' Available from: https://researchbriefings.files.parliament.uk/documents/CBP-7626/CBP-7626.pdf

Wang, H.J., et al. (2010). Alcohol, inflammation, and gut-liver-brain interactions in tissue damage and disease development. Available from: https://www.ncbi.nlm.nih.gov/pmc/articles/PMC2842521/

Cirino, E. (2023). Why does alcohol make me bloated? Available from: https://www.healthline.com/health/alcohol-bloating

Butts, M., et al. (2023). The Influence of Alcohol Consumption on Intestinal Nutrient Absorption: A Comprehensive Review. Available from: https://www.ncbi.nlm.nih.gov/pmc/articles/PMC10096942/

Brady, C.W. (2015) Liver disease in menopause. Available from: https://www.ncbi.nlm.nih.gov/pmc/articles/PMC4491951/

Fielding, S. (2024). How much do genetics influence the aging process? Available from: https://mcpress.mayoclinic.org/healthy-aging/how-much-do-genetics-influence-the-aging-process/

Centers for Disease Control and Prevention. (2024). Epigenetics, Health, and Disease. Available from: https://www.cdc.gov/genomics-and-health/about/epigenetic-impacts-on-health.html

Nikolis, A., and Enright, K.M. (2021). A Multicenter Evaluation of Paradoxical Adipose Hyperplasia Following Cryolipolysis for Fat Reduction and Body Contouring: A Review of 8658 Cycles in 2114 Patients. Available from: https://pubmed.ncbi.nlm.nih.gov/33216910/

Li, W., Seo, I., Kim, B., Fassih, A., Southall, M., & Parsa, R. (2021). Low-level red plus near infrared lights combination induces expressions of collagen and elastin in human skin in vitro. Available from: https://pubmed.ncbi.nlm.nih.gov/33594706/

# THE NON-SURGICAL SKIN REVOLUTION

A Beauty Studio Medi Spa production
bsmedispa.co.uk

Printed in Great Britain
by Amazon